Aids to Obstetrics and Gynaecology

Other titles in the Aids series

Badenoch Aids to Urology
Benn Aids to Microbiology and Infectious Diseases
Burton Aids to Postgraduate Medicine 5E
Burton Aids to Undergraduate Medicine 4E
Child Aids to Clinical Haematology
Dixon Aids to Pathology 3E
Habel Aids to Paediatrics 2E
Habel Aids to Paediatrics for Undergraduates
Hayes et al Aids to Gastroenterology and Hepatology
Hayes and MacWalter Aids to Clinical Examination
Hornsby and Winter Aids to Part 1 FRCP
Khaw et al Aids to Ophthalmology
Lee Aids to Physiotherapy 2E
MacMahon Aids to Paediatric Surgery
Mead Aids to General Practice
Moore-Gillon and Stafford Aids to ENT
Morgan Aids to Psychiatry 3E
Mowschenson Aids to Undergraduate Surgery 3E
Muirhead and Catto Aids to Fluid and Electrolyte Balance
Patterson-Brown and Eckersley Aids to Anatomy
Poston Aids to Operative Surgery
Reynolds and Freeman Aids to Clinical Chemistry
Rogers and Spector Aids to Clinical Pharmacology and Therapeutics 2E
Rogers and Spector Aids to Pharmacology 2E
Scratcherd Aids to Physiology 3E
Sinclair and Webb Aids to Undergraduate Obstetrics and Gynaecology
Stevenson and Chahal Aids to Endocrinology
Stirrat Aids to Reproductive Biology
Watkins and Thomas Aids to Postgraduate Surgery 3E
Weir Aids to Immunology

For Churchill Livingstone:
Publisher: Peter Richardson
Design: Design Resources Unit
Production: Neil Dickson
Editorial Co-ordination: Editorial Resources Unit
Copy Editor: Paul Singleton
Indexer: Laurence Errington
Sales Promotion Executive: Louise Johnstone

Aids to Obstetrics and Gynaecology

For MRCOG

Gordon M. Stirrat

MA MD FRCOG

Professor of Obstetrics and Gynaecology
University of Bristol

THIRD EDITION

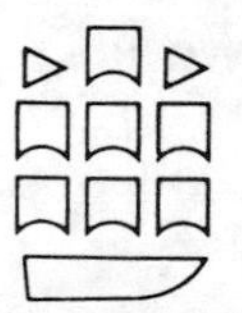

CHURCHILL LIVINGSTONE
EDINBURGH LONDON MELBOURNE NEW YORK AND TOKYO 1991

CHURCHILL LIVINGSTONE
Medical Division of Longman Group UK Limited

Distributed in the United States of America by Churchill Livingstone Inc., 650 Avenue of the Americas, New York, 10011, and by associated companies, branches and representatives throughout the world.

First edition 1983
Second edition 1987
Third edition 1991
Reprinted 1992

ISBN 0-443-04382-5

British Library Cataloguing in Publication Data
Stirrat, Gordon M.
Aids to obstetrics and gynaecology: For MRCOG
— 3rd ed.— (Aids)
I. Title II. Series
618

Library of Congress Cataloging in Publication Data
Stirrat, Gordon M.
Aids to obstetrics and gynecology: for MRCOG/Gordon M.
Stirrat — 3rd ed.
p. cm. — (Aids series)
Key elements of Aids to reproductive biology have been incorporated.
Includes bibliographical references and index.
ISBN 0-443-04382-5
1. Gynecology — Outlines, syllabi, etc. 2. Obstetrics — Outlines, syllabi, etc. I. Stirrat, Gordon M. Aids to reproductive biology.
II. Title. III. Series: Aids (Series) (Edinburgh, Scotland)
[DNLM: 1. Gynecology — outlines. 2. Obstetrics — outlines. WQ 18 S861ab]
RG112.S75 1991
618 — dc20
DNLM/DLC
for Library of Congress 91–386
CIP

Produced by Longman Singapore Publishers (Pte) Ltd
Printed in Singapore

The publisher's policy is to use **paper manufactured from sustainable forests**

Preface to the third edition

This third edition has been produced with the same aims as the first and as complete a revision as the second. Key elements of *Aids to Reproductive Biology* have also been incorporated to make it a cohesive whole.

Once more, progress in knowledge and practice has required significant alterations and changes of emphasis. In this I have been considerably assisted by my friends and colleagues Peter Fleming, David James, Ruth Skrine and Peter Wardle. As ever, any residual errors are mine. I am very grateful to Mrs Pam Hendry for typing the revised text. I am also grateful to Churchill Livingstone for continuing to give me the opportunity to be involved in the teaching of others. I hope that what I have written will be of as much help to them as that of my teachers has been to me.

Bristol, 1991 G.M.S.

Preface to the first edition

This book aims to provide a synoptic guide to the essentials of clinical obstetrics and gynaecology. It and its companion volume *Aids to Reproductive Biology* have been written primarily with candidates for Parts 1 and 2 of the MRCOG in mind. It is hoped, however, that others will find them helpful also.

Within the constraints of size and its synoptic nature it is as comprehensive and up-to-date as possible. The validity of other viewpoints is acknowledged and the reader is encouraged to supplement his knowledge from among the books in the suggested further reading lists.

It is not possible to divorce pathology from physiology and this volume contains clinically important elements of both. Further valuable information on general pathology can be obtained from another title in this series — *Aids to Pathology* by M. F. Dixon. The work of a multitude of eminent authors and the example of a series of outstanding teachers has contributed to the body of knowledge summarised here. I am more grateful than I can express to two great men (Professor Ian Donald and Professor Alec Turnbull) who have influenced my career, philosophy and attitudes more than they will ever know.

Finally, I wish yet again to acknowledge especially the work of Mrs Betty French, not only for typing the manuscript but also for keeping me in order over the past six years.

Bristol, 1983 G.M.S.

Contents

SECTION ONE

Obstetrics

Obstetric care

OBSTETRIC CARE

Obstetric care has four phases:
1. Pre-conception (p. 4)
2. Antenatal (p. 5)
3. Intrapartum (p. 119)
4. Postnatal (p. 156)

Its objectives are:
1. *Risk assessment* — to assess risk of harm to mother and baby
2. *Counselling* — to (i) advise the mother and her partner about the nature and extent of any perceived risks, and (ii) advise on how to minimise or eradicate the effects of any risk factors
3. *Education* — to (i) provide continuing education on normal pregnancy and childbirth for the mother and her partner, and (ii) give some guidance about pregnancy problems and possible interventions
4. *Treatment* — to treat any condition which might affect, or be affected by, the pregnancy
5. *Satisfaction* — to make the pregnancy and delivery as fulfilling yet as safe as possible

RISK AND PREGNANCY

Risk is the probability that a particular event will occur. An 'at risk' pregnancy is one in which the probability of an adverse outcome in the mother and/or baby is greater than that for pregnant women in general. A high risk of one particular outcome does not necessarily imply a high risk of other adverse outcomes. For the terms 'high risk' and 'low risk' to be useful, the probability, nature and extent of specific risks must be considered. A low risk of a serious condition with a bad outcome should be given more weight than a high risk of a lesser problem which has minor effects. Factors associated with risk of a particular event are 'risk markers'. Perception of risk varies among individuals, e.g. a stated chance of 95% for a good outcome (e.g. chromosomally normal baby) may be perceived as good news. The identical 5% risk of having a baby with Down's syndrome is often thought to be bad news. A guide to the extent of particular risks in pregnancy (e.g. pre-term birth, intrauterine growth retardation, congenital malformation or perinatal death) can be obtained from:

1. History and examination for presence of risk markers
2. *Screening tests* offered to all pregnant women (see p. 39).
   For a screening test to be of value it must:
   (i) Predict the great majority of those who have the condition (*high positive predictive power*)
   (ii) Exclude those who do not have the condition (*high negative predictive power*)
   All screening tests have some *false-positive* and *false-negative* results. The clinical value depends on the balance between them and the severity of the condition. A test of value when the incidence of a condition is high will be of poorer predictive value in another population with a low incidence of the same condition
3. *Diagnostic tests* for those in whom a screening test is positive, or who have clinical signs and symptoms

Interventions
Diagnostic and therapeutic interventions have their own intrinsic risk. On some occasions an intervention may cause the harm one is trying to prevent. An intervention without proven benefit cannot be justified on the basis that it will 'do no harm'.

PRE-CONCEPTION CARE

It is important that care begins *before* pregnancy because:

1. Many women enter pregnancy poorly nourished, smoking heavily, and in a less than optimal state of health
2. The most critical phase of fetal development is complete by the time of the first antenatal clinic attendance, and adverse factors have already begun to produce their effects

Pre-conception clinics allow:

1. Women with chronic diseases to become pregnant in as healthy a condition as possible
2. Dietary advice to be offered to those above or below ideal body weight
3. Encouragement to give up smoking and reduce alcohol ingestion
4. Advice to be given to those who are anxious, have had problems in a previous pregnancy, or who have a personal or family history of a congenitally malformed child

5. Rubella immunisation to be offered if the woman is susceptible
6. Baseline measures of weight and blood pressure to be obtained

Much of this care is the proper responsibility of the primary health care team; however, obstetricians, physicians, and clinical geneticists should be prepared to provide the benefit of their expertise.

ANTENATAL CARE

Antenatal care is a screening system which aims to assess and obviate risk of harm to mother and baby. Traditional patterns of care were established over 50 years ago; their primary objective was to reduce maternal mortality and morbidity. Few of the measures used routinely have been evaluated in the context of today's most pressing problems.

Booking clinic

The woman should be seen by her general practitioner early (usually within the first 8 weeks) in pregnancy. Assessment of risk begins there. The first hospital booking visit should take place between 12 and 16 weeks' gestation.

ROUTINE BOOKING ASSESSMENT

Administrative details, including age, marital status, and gravidity, are recorded. An accurate menstrual history is important.

History	Medical and surgical; obstetric; family; social, smoking, alcohol and drug ingestion; inoculation risk (see p. 100)
Examination	Weight; height; blood pressure; urinalysis for protein, blood and glucose General — chest, heart, breasts, etc Abdominal — masses, tenderness, fundal height Pelvic — routine vaginal examination is unnecessary Cervical smear if none within past 5 years Ultrasound scan (see p. 10)
Investigations	FBC and check for haemoglobinopathy when indicated (see p. 34); ABO and Rh group and check for antibodies Rubella immunity; VDRL AFP at 16 to 18 weeks' (optional); hepatitis B status; HIV status in women at high risk (see p. 101) with their consent Screen for toxoplasmosis if at high risk (see p. 104) MSU for culture and sensitivity Chest X-ray (if at high risk of tuberculosis)

The appropriate pattern of antenatal care and place of delivery can now be determined based on the risk factors which have been discovered. The policy must be continually re-appraised during pregnancy.

Markers associated with risk of adverse outcome to baby and/or mother

Marker	*Nature of adverse outcome*	*Mechanism*
1. *Social factors*		
Teenage pregnancy	Increase in risk of pre-term birth, small-for-dates babies, perinatal and infant death (particularly due to SIDS)	Linked to socio-economic factors — illegitimacy, poor housing and social environment, poor education, lack of support, and smoking
Maternal age ≥35 years	Increase in risk of Down Syndrome (see p. 31); other risks not greatly increased	Unknown
Maternal age ≥40 years	As above, and rate of pre-eclampsia, pre-term and precipitate labour, and malpresentation increased; perinatal and maternal mortality raised	Partly linked to socio-economic factors and parity effects; age itself also has some effect
Primigravidity	Pre-eclampsia is an 'unknown' quantity in reproductive terms	Unknown
High parity and low inter-pregnancy interval	Increased rate of miscarriage; perinatal and maternal morbidity; twinning; congenital malformations, hypertension and APH	Socio-economic and nutritional factors; associated with smoking effects
Poor social conditions	All risks increased	
Smoking 10 or more cigarettes/day (see p. 55)	Increased rate of IUGR, perinatal and infant mortality; rate of pre-eclampsia reduced but effects more severe	General toxic effects of tobacco products
Heavy drinking (>80 g alcohol/day) (see p. 55)	Fetal alcohol syndrome with mental retardation; pre-term labour, perinatal and maternal mortality	Direct effects of alcohol plus general socio-economic effects and smoking

Marker	*Nature of adverse outcome*	*Mechanism*
Drug abuse (see p. 55)	Increased rate of miscarriage, IUGR, perinatal, infant and maternal mortality, pre-term delivery, hepatitis and HIV infections (if IV drug abuser)	Socio-economic effects, malnutrition, direct drug effects and infection
2. *Physical factors*		
Height 1.54 m or less	Dysfunctional labour and need for instrumental delivery	Pelvic capacity
More than 10% over ideal body weight	Risk of diabetes, hypertension increased	Metabolic effects
3. *Genetic factors*		
Family history of diabetes in first-degree relative	Gestational diabetes	Metabolic 'stress' of pregnancy
Family or personal history of other inheritable diseases (e.g. haemoglobinopathy)	Risk depends on nature of inheritance of condition	See relevant sections
Congenital malformations in mother, family or previous child		
4. *Medical factors*		
Medical disorders (e.g. anaemia auto-immune, cardiac, renal or endocrine disease	Risk depends on nature and severity of condition	See relevant sections
Past history of thrombo-embolism	Risk of recurrence	Damaged venous endothelium with increased coagulation factors in pregnancy
Rhesus negative with antibodies	Iso-immunisation with fetal anaemia	Immunological
5. *Obstetric factors*		
Previous pre-term delivery	Increased risk of recurrence	'Idiopathic'; cervical incompetence; uterine anomaly
Elevated serum AFP with NTD	IUGR, perinatal morbidity and mortality	Unknown
Previous low birthweight infant (<2.5 kg)	Risk of recurrence	Genetic predisposition to small babies; 'placental insufficiency'

Marker	*Nature of adverse outcome*	*Mechanism*
Previous large baby (>4.0 kg)	Risk of recurrence; birth trauma; shoulder dystocia; C-P disproportion	Genetic predisposition (impaired glucose tolerance?)
Previous stillbirth or neonatal death	Risk of recurrence	Varies with cause
Multiple pregnancy	Rates of miscarriage, pre-term delivery, pre-eclampsia, anaemia, antepartum haemorrhage, perinatal and maternal mortality increased	Various
Previous Caesarean section	Maternal and perinatal mortality; recurrence of dysfunctional labour	Dehiscence of scar
Previous placental abruption or third stage abnormality	Risk of recurrence	
Previous third degree tear	Recurrent damage to anal sphincter	Direct trauma
6. *Gynaecological factors*		
Involuntary infertility and recurrent miscarriage	Miscarriage, perinatal mortality, IUGR, pre-eclampsia (poor pregnancy outcome in general)	Related to maternal age, otherwise unknown (see relevant section)
Previous myomectomy	Risk not great	Related to maternal age and infertility
Fibroids	Miscarriage; malpresentation; IUGR	Implantation site
Cone biopsy	Cervical dystocia	Fibrosis
Pelvic floor repair	Further damage to pelvic floor during vaginal delivery	Direct trauma
7. *Psychological factors*		
Recent divorce, separation or major family upset	Pre-term delivery	Unknown
Previous or current depression or other serious psychiatric disorder	Worsening in pregnancy or puerperium; harm to self or baby	Hormonal?

Women at low risk of pregnancy problems can be delivered by their own midwife and GP. The ideal criteria for booking in a GP unit isolated from a maternity hospital or for home confinement are:

1. Second, third or fourth pregnancy under 35 years of age
2. No medical, psychological or obstetric contra-indications
3. No rhesus or other antibodies

Criteria may not need to be so strict when GP and consultant until are integrated: individual cases can be discussed among the mother, the midwife and GP, and the hospital team.

CONTINUING ANTENATAL CARE

The traditional pattern of care involves the woman being seen by a midwife and/or doctor every 4 weeks to 28 weeks; every 2 weeks from 28 to 36 weeks, and weekly thereafter. This has not been proven to be necessary in women at low risk of developing complications for whom the following schedule is suggested, shared between GP and hospital:

8 to 12 weeks	to GP to arrange booking and confirm dates	
16 weeks	to consultant, hospital or peripheral clinic for booking, serology and screening tests (e.g. ultrasound, serum AFP)	
26 or 28 weeks	to check fetal growth	with GP/midwife
36 weeks	to check presentation	
40 weeks	pre-delivery assessment	
41 weeks	to hospital if not delivered	

Any additional visits should have a clearly specified objective, e.g. risk markers now present.

ROUTINE ASSESSMENTS

Every subsequent visit:
- Urinalysis
- Blood pressure
- Exclude peripheral oedema
- Measure and record fundal height (in centimetres above symphysis pubis)

Every visit in third trimester:
- Fetal lie and presentation
- Presence of fetal heart
- Record patient awareness of fetal movement

At 26 and 36 weeks (as a minimum):
- Full blood count
- Rh-D antibodies in Rh negative women and other antibodies if necessary

The presence (or development) of adverse features demands closer attention than above and the introduction of more sophisticated methods of assessment of maternal and fetal welfare (see pp. 45–52). Among the risk markers which can arise during pregnancy are:

Vaginal bleeding	Oligohydramnios
Hypertension	Marked reduction in fetal movements in last trimester
Proteinuria	
Persistent glycosuria	IUGR as assessed by deviation from normal growth of the uterine fundus or by ultrasound (p. 47)
Urinary tract or other infections	
Polyhydramnios	Malpresentations (after 34 weeks)

ULTRASOUND IN ANTENATAL CARE

Among the clinical situations in which ultrasonic examination is most useful are:

1. Assessment of vaginal bleeding and/or abdominal pain in early pregnancy
2. Accurate ascertainment of gestational age — menstrual history can be unreliable in up to 45% of women
3. Allowing more exact interpretation of serum AFP levels
4. Exclusion of multiple pregnancy
5. Examination of the fetus when risk of congenital anomaly is high and before amniocentesis or chorionic villus sampling
6. To check fetal size and liquor volume when the uterus is small or large for dates
7. Monitoring fetal growth in high-risk pregnancies
8. Ascertaining the placental site and identifying the source of any APH
9. Determination of fetal presentation if it is unclear by palpation
10. Discovering fetal attitude in malpresentation
11. More confident timing of any obstetric intervention (e.g. for postmaturity)

The performance of a routine scan at 16–18 weeks' gestation is common. Although it cannot be shown significantly to affect outcome, it is generally considered to be of value. A second routine scan at 32 to 36 weeks is not indicated in the absence of any risk markers.

Safety of ultrasound

There is no evidence that ultrasound is anything but safe for mother, baby and operator (see Suggested further reading). The skill of the operator is of prime importance. Misleading information will lead to wrong management decisions.

OTHER ASPECTS OF CARE

This is an important time to provide health education and advice on, for example, diet, dental care, smoking (avoid it), coitus (no association with adverse pregnancy outcome) and maternity benefits.

Preparation for labour and breast-feeding should begin well in advance.

SUGGESTED FURTHER READING

Enkin M, Chalmers I (eds) 1982 Effectiveness and satisfaction in antenatal care. Spastics International Medical Publications, London
Enkin M, Kierse M J N C, Chalmers I (eds) 1989 Effective care in pregnancy and childbirth. Oxford University Press, Oxford
James D K, Stirrat G M 1988 Pregnancy and risk. Wiley, Chichester
Report of RCOG Working Party on routine ultrasound examination in pregnancy 1989 RCOG, London
Turnbull A, Chamberlain G (eds) 1989 Obstetrics. Churchill Livingstone, Edinburgh

Early pregnancy and its disorders

FERTILISATION AND IMPLANTATION

Male and female fertility is discussed on pp. 183–186.

1. *Fertilisation.* At ovulation the ovum is deposited near the fimbrial end of the Fallopian tube and enters the tube due to the fimbrial ciliated epithelium. Of the millions of sperm deposited in the vagina, only a few thousand enter the Fallopian tubes, and of these only a few hundred reach the ovum. Fertilisation usually takes place in the ampulla (i.e. outer third) of the tube. Many sperm pierce the zona pellucida to enter the *perivitelline space*, but only one sperm can pierce the *vitelline membrane.* The whole spermatozoon is engulfed, but the neck and tail become detached from the head and disintegrate. The head forms the *male pronucleus.* Penetration of the vitelline membrane causes the second meiotic division of the oocyte to be completed. The second polar body is extruded into the perivitelline space. The ovum is now termed the *female pronucleus.* The male and female pronuclei fuse to form the zygote and restore the normal diploid number of chromosomes.
2. *Formation of the blastocyst.* The zygote becomes the morula and then the blastocyst by repeated cell division. The morula differentiates into two cell groups:
   - (i) The *trophoblast,* which invades the uterine wall and establishes the placenta (95% of the cells of the morula)
   - (ii) The *embryoblast* (5% of the cells) which produces all the tissues of the embryo from three different cellular layers — the ectoderm, the mesoderm and the endoderm
3. *Implantation and development of the placenta.* Implantation depends on a complex series of signals which pass between the invading cytotrophoblast and cells of and within the endometrium (see Suggested further reading). The blastocyst always implants at its *embryonic pole* where embryoblast meets trophoblast. Implantation occurs on the posterior wall in about two-thirds of cases and on the anterior wall in about one-third of cases. The timetable is as follows:

Event	*Time from fertilisation*
First cleavage	30 hours
Second cleavage	40 hours
Morula formed (16-cell stage to formation of blasctocyst)	50 to 60 hours
Morula reaches uterus and blastocyst forms (from 50- to 60-cell stage)	4 to 5 days
Implantation begins	7 days
Implantation is complete	14 days
Primary, secondary then tertiary villi form sequentially	12 to 16 days
Fetal circulation becomes established	21 to 28 days

detect fetal heart by 6/40 (USS)

SUGGESTED FURTHER READING

Dewhurst J, de Swiet M, Chamberlain G V P 1986 Basic science in obstetrics and gynaecology. Churchill Livingstone, Edinburgh
Johnson M, Everitt B 1988 Essential reproduction. Blackwell Scientific, Oxford
Mastroianni L, Coutifaris C 1990 The FIGO manual of human reproduction, vol 1, reproductive physiology. Parthenon, Carnforth

ABORTION

Definition

1. Biological — the expulsion or extraction of products of conception before fetal viability is achieved.
2. Epidemiological (WHO) — the expulsion or extraction from its mother of an embryo or fetus weighing 500 g or less.

Any fetus delivered and 'showing signs of life' becomes a potential live birth and should be registered as such.

Spontaneous abortion (miscarriage)

Incidence

The loss rate among clinically recognised pregnancies is about 15%. It may rise to 50% if unrecognised pregnancies are included. Most occur within the first 14 weeks.

Potential causes

1. No demonstrable cause — this is the commonest situation
2. Chromosomes anomalies may cause up to 25% of all miscarriages, particularly trisomy, XO and triploidy
3. 'Blighted ovum', anembryonic pregnancy, abnormality of placental development

4. Multiple pregnancy
5. Uterine — e.g. congenital or acquired cervical incompetence; congenital uterine anomalies; subserous fibroids
6. Corpus luteum failure — it is more likely that the corpus luteum is failing because abortion is occurring rather than the converse; an increased miscarriage rate among women with polycystic ovary disease may relate to corpus luteum failure (see p. 17)
7. Infections, e.g. rubella, cytomegalovirus, any acute pyrexial illness or condition causing peritonitis
8. 'Immunological'? (see below)

Threatened abortion

The features are:
1. Amenorrhoea followed by slight vaginal bleeding
2. No pain
3. The uterus is the correct size for dates
4. The cervix is closed

If an ultrasonic scan can demonstrate a fetal heart there is a 90% chance that the pregnancy will progress satisfactorily.

Bed rest is of no therapeutic value, and treatment with progestogens or hCG cannot be justified.

Inevitable (incomplete) abortion

The features are:
1. Amenorrhoea followed by heavy vaginal bleeding
2. Pain follows bleeding (cf. ectopic pregnancy)
3. The uterus may be small, large or correct size for dates
4. The cervix is dilating and products of conception may be passing through the os

Give ergometrine 0.5 mg i.m. and arrange evacuation of the uterus. If the uterus is larger than 12 weeks' size set up syntocinon infusion to cause reduction in uterine size before undertaking evacuation.

Complete abortion

The features are:
1. Amenorrhoea followed by a variable amount of bleeding which has now stopped
2. The uterus is smaller than expected
3. The cervix is closed

It is common practice to carry out exploration of the uterus lest some products are retained. An ultrasonic scan (especially if a vaginal transducer is used) showing an empty uterine cavity may help to prevent unnecessary surgical procedures.

Missed abortion

Retention of the products of conception after death of the embryo or fetus.

The features are:

1. Amenorrhoea during which an episode of slight vaginal bleeding may or may not have occurred
2. Regression of earlier signs and symptoms of pregnancy
3. Uterus small-for-dates
4. The cervix is closed
5. Ultrasonic examination either shows a collapsed gestation sac or fails to detect a fetal heart or movements

If left alone, resorption or spontaneous expulsion will occur but it is best to proceed to evacuate the uterus in most cases once a firm diagnosis has been made.

Management

Uterus at or less than 12 weeks' size — proceed to careful suction aspiration of uterus under GA.

Uterus greater than 12 weeks' size — use vaginal or extra-amniotic prostaglandins to induce abortion. Subsequent evacuation may be necessary.

Septic abortion

An incomplete abortion complicated by infection of the uterine contents. This may be due to criminal interference.

The features are as for incomplete abortion accompanied by pyrexia (⩾38°C) and tachycardia, general malaise, abdominal pain, marked pelvic tenderness and purulent vaginal loss. Other causes of an 'acute abdomen' and generalized infection must be excluded.

Pathogenesis

The commonest infection organisms are: *E. coli* (and other Gram-negative bacteria), streptococci (haemolytic and anaerobic), other anaerobes (e.g. *Bacteroides*) and *Staphylococcus*. Although infections with *Cl. perfringens* and *Cl. tetani* are infrequent now they are potentially lethal if not treated promptly and adequately.

Pathology

The infection is usually mild (80%) being confined to the decidua but it can spread to the myometrium and beyond (15%). In the remainder (5%) more generalised signs and symptoms appear due to the release of endotoxins (see below). Endotoxic shock and disseminated intravascular coagulation may develop in these severe cases.

Investigation
Take cervical swabs for bacteriology in all cases and blood cultures if the pyrexia is at or greater than 38.4°C.

In severe infections monitor fluid and electrolyte balance and check coagulation status.

Management

1. *Antibiotic therapy* — for mild cases give a broad-spectrum antibiotic and metronidazole orally while awaiting the results of bacteriology cultures.

   In moderate and severe cases the intravenous route is preferred but metronidazole can be given rectally
2. *Evacuation of the uterus* — this is probably better deferred until reasonable tissue levels of antibiotics have been achieved (i.e. about 12 hours). The timing of intervention may of course be dictated by other circumstances

Recurrent miscarriage

Definition
Three or more consecutive miscarriages. Primary recurrent miscarriage — all pregnancies have ended in loss. Secondary recurrent miscarriage — one (usually the first) pregnancy has proceeded to viability with all others ending in loss.

Incidence
Less than 1% of women of reproductive age.

Clinical management of recurrent miscarriage

Associated Factor	*Investigation and Diagnosis*	*Treatment*	*Comment*
1. *Anatomical disorders*			
(i) Uterine abnormalities	Hysterosalpingogram (HSG) or vaginal ultrasound	A septum can be divided by utriculoplasty or vaginally using an operating hysteroscope	Abdominal operation can cause infertility
(ii) Fibroids	Hysterosalpingogram (HSG) or vaginal ultrasound	Myomectomy	True role of fibroids unclear
(iii) Ascherman's syndrome (intrauterine synechiae)	Hysteroscopy	Division of synechiae	Usually caused by multiple curettage
(iv) Cervical incompetence,	HSG or vaginal ultrasound	Cervical cerclage	True diagnosis difficult and

Associated Factor	Investigation and Diagnosis	Treatment	Comment
congenital or acquired			benefit from treatment uncertain
2. *Genetic disorders*			
(i) Recurrent aneuploidy	Fetal karyotyping	None — occurs as a chance event or related to maternal age	Sporadic genetic disorders recurring consecutively by chance may explain many recurrent miscarriages
(ii) Parental balanced translocation	Parental karyotypes	Genetic counselling (see p. 38)	Accounts for 4% of cases
(iii) Molecular mutations	DNA analysis may be available in the future		Speculative
3. *Endocrine factors*			
(i) Inadequate luteal phase	Luteal phase <10 days; progesterone levels <15 nmol/l in five consecutive cycles; endometrial biopsy(?)	Clomiphene, progesterone or hCG (empirical treatment not justified)	Reported incidence varies between 3 and 60%
(ii) Polycystic ovary disease	See p. 175	See p. 177	May have a small role in recurrent losses
(iii) Thyroid function	Not justified	Not justified	Not a cause
(iv) Diabetes	Not justified	Not justified	Not a cause
4. *Reproductive tract infections* Few data exist to support infection as a cause of recurrent pregnancy loss. Well-designed studies are necessary.			
5. *Immunological causes*			
(i) Anti-cardiolipin (ACA) syndrome	Check APTT routinely in all cases; carry out more detailed auto-immune screen and check specifically for anti-cardiolipin antibodies and lupus inhibitor if indicated (see p. 87)	Low dose aspirin and/or steroids for women with ACA syndrome (see p. 87); *not* justified empirically	Tends to be associated with secondary recurrent miscarriage

Clinical management of recurrent miscarriage

Associated Factor	*Investigation and Diagnosis*	*Treatment*	*Comment*
(ii) Disorders of materno–fetal immune status	None routinely	The benefit of immuno-therapy is not yet proven	Scientific basis for investigation and therapy not strong
6. *Psychological causes*	?	'Tender loving care'	Evidence for this is no better and no worse than for several other 'causes'

Even after three consecutive losses the spontaneous chance of a successful pregnancy is over 60%. The success of all 'treatments' needs to be viewed with the spontaneous success rate in mind.

When the woman with a history of repeated miscarriages becomes pregnant she requires careful antenatal supervision.

Poor reproductive performance tends also to be reflected in an increased incidence of other pregnancy complications.

SUGGESTED FURTHER READING

Bennett M J, Edmonds D K 1987 Spontaneous and recurrent abortion. Blackwell Scientific, Oxford

Oakley A, McPherson A, Roberts H 1984 Miscarriage. Fontana, London

Turnbull A, Chamberlain G (eds) 1989 Obstetrics. Churchill Livingstone, Edinburgh

ECTOPIC PREGNANCY

Definition

The implantation of a pregnancy outside the uterine cavity.

Incidence

About 10 to 12/1000 pregnancies with increased risk

— among black women in USA (20/1000)

— in West Indies (30/1000)

— in age range 25 to 34 years (comprise 65% of ectopics)

It causes over 10% of all maternal deaths and is the commonest cause of first-trimester deaths. Two-thirds of deaths are due to delay in diagnosis and treatment and, therefore, potentially preventable. After one ectopic the risk of recurrence is between 10 and 20%.

Sites of ectopic pregnancies

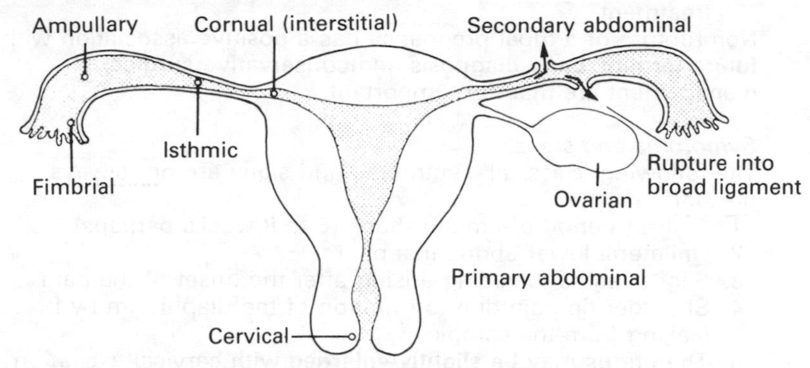

The incidence of heterotopic pregnancies (i.e. a combination of intra- and extrauterine) is about 1:30 000. It has increased with greater use of assisted conception techniques.

Tubal pregnancy (95%)

Predisposing factors:

1. Maternal age — there has been a tendency to postpone pregnancy to the age range of greatest risk
2. Congenital — e.g. tubal diverticula
3. Pelvic inflammatory disease (PID) impedes the progress of the ovum/zygote due to adhesions, fimbrial agglutination, tubal narrowing or destruction of the cilia of the endosalpinx, but no evidence of PID can be found in 50% of cases
4. Tubal surgery
5. Intrauterine devices prevent intrauterine pregnancy effectively, tubal implantation to a lesser extent, and ovarian pregnancy not at all; the relative rate of ectopic pregnancies therefore increases
6. Progestogen contraceptives may be associated with a higher incidence because the drug reduces tubal motility and, if conception occurs, it is more likely to lodge in the tube
7. Previous tubal pregnancy
8. Assisted conception (particularly IVF) if tubes are patent and damaged

Consequences of tubal implantation

Without intervention, the following would happen:

1. The conceptus dies and is gradually reabsorbed
2. The conceptus is aborted from the tube into the peritoneal cavity; this is the most common outcome. Rarely the conceptus may still be viable and a secondary abdominal pregnancy ensues (see below)

3. The tube ruptures and bleeding occurs, requiring emergency treatment

Non-rupture of a tubal pregnancy has a positive association with future fertility. Early diagnosis and conservative surgical management are therefore important.

Symptoms and signs

The following 'classical' symptoms and signs are not always present:

1. A short period of amenorrhoea (6 to 8 weeks perhaps)
2. Unilateral lower abdominal pain
3. Slight vaginal bleeding arising after the onset of the pain
4. Shoulder tip pain due to irritation of the diaphragm by blood leaking from the ectopic
5. The uterus may be slightly enlarged with cervical excitation and tenderness
6. A small tender mass may be palpable to one side of the uterus. *N.B.* If the history is strongly suggestive of an ectopic pregnancy DO NOT carry out a vaginal examination unless rapid access can be gained to an operating theatre. The tube may rupture, the patient being put at severe risk.

Diagnosis

The diagnosis is not made in 20 to 25% of cases. Even when it is, the presentation-to-treatment interval is over 48 hours in 40 to 50%, and over 1 week in 20 to 25%.

Differential diagnosis

1. Threatened or incomplete abortion. In the former there is no pain and in the latter pain follows vaginal bleeding
2. Bleeding corpus luteum — laparoscopy is required to make this differentiation
3. Accident to an ovarian cyst — there is usually no menstrual delay. Laparoscopy is indicated
4. Pelvic inflammation — the systemic reaction is more profound and the signs are usually bilateral

Appropriate intervention must be based on index of suspicion — 'think ectopic'.

Investigation

For women in clinically stable conditions with no evidence of intra-abdominal bleeding:

1. *B-hCG estimations — urine*. The latex agglutination inhibition tests are not sensitive enough. Newer monoclonal antibody immunoenzymatic dip-stick assays detect hCG at a level of 1 i.u./l and are therefore useful
   Serum — a negative result virtually excludes an ectopic

pregnancy, but maintain suspicion if other clinical features are suggestive.
If the urine or serum test is positive but neither an intra- nor extrauterine pregnancy can be confirmed by ultrasound, repeat test in 48 h.
The levels of hCG rise more slowly when the pregnancy is extrauterine

2. *Ultrasound*. This aids diagnosis by:
   (i) Demonstrating an intrauterine pregnancy with no other pelvic pathology; the fetal node must be observed — a pseudogestational sac can cause confusion. A normal intrauterine pregnancy becomes visible by abdominal transducer at about 6 weeks, and earlier using a transvaginal transducer (5/40)
   (ii) Visualising an ectopic, (best using transvaginal approach), or complex cystic adnexal masses
   (iii) Demonstrating free fluid (blood) in abdomen
3. *Laparoscopy*. This is the gold standard for diagnosis and is indicated if index of suspicion is high. *Very early tubal pregnancies* (3 to 4% of total) *can still be missed at laparoscopy*

Management of acute situation
If the patient is shocked, laparotomy must be undertaken as quickly as possible. The priorities are to stop haemorrhage a prevent further bleeding. Conservative surgery is less likely to be possible under these circumstances.

Surgical approach if tube unruptured
1. *Laparotomy* — this is still the most commonly used approach. Conservative surgery should be attempted if that is what the woman wishes. *Routine salpingectomy is to be deprecated*
   Procedures:
   1. Try to milk the pregnancy from the tube, or
   2. Carry out a linear salpingostomy along the anti-mesenteric border. The tubal incision can be left open or can be closed in one or two layers by 6/0 sutures
2. *Operative laparoscopy*. This technique requires more skill and expertise than is generally available at present
   Potential benefits:
   (i) May reduce adhesion formation
   (ii) Reduces postoperative stay and convalescence
   Potential hazards:
   (i) Delayed haemorrhage
   (ii) Continued trophoblast growth

Comp

Indications:
Unruptured ampullary or infundibular pregnancy less than 3 cm in diameter with no bleeding into peritoneal cavity
Contra-indications:
(i) Absolute — shock
(ii) Relative — tubal rupture; haemoperitoneum; pelvic adhesions; tube more than 3 cm in diameter; concurrent medical problems
Procedures:
Linear salpingostomy can be carried out and closed or left open as above. (For technique see Suggested further reading.) Partial or complete salpingectomy is also possible

Serial hCG levels must be followed postoperatively to exclude persistent trophoblast growth.

Cornual pregnancy
This uncommon form of ectopic pregnancy can have serious consequences because it is difficult to diagnose early, and when it ruptures it is associated with profuse intraperitoneal bleeding. Injection of methotrexate into the sac under ultrasound guidance has been reported.

Ovarian pregnancy
To make a diagnosis of primary ovarian pregnancy the following three features must be present:
1. The fallopian tube must be intact
2. The gestation sac must occupy the anatomical site of the ovary
3. Ovarian tissue must be demonstrable histologically in the specimen

Abdominal pregnancy
Both primary and secondary abdominal pregnancies are rare events. The fetus may develop fully and survive but the woman usually presents as an acute abdominal emergency in the second trimester.

It may be possible to make a prospective correct diagnosis if the following features are borne in mind:
1. There is often a history of an episode of abdominal pain and slight vaginal bleeding early in pregnancy which settled
2. Maternal serum AFP may be elevated
3. The ultrasound scan shows oligohydramnios and no clear uterine outline around the sac. There is also a separate mass related to the gestation sac (this is the uterus)

When laparotomy is carried out it may not be possible or advisable to remove the placenta because it is likely to be fixed to the abdominal viscera.

Cervical pregnancy

This is also rare but may cause profuse vaginal bleeding. Hysterectomy may be necessary. Injection of methotrexate into the sac is an alternative if the diagnosis is made early enough.

SUGGESTED FURTHER READING

Macafee C J 1984 Ectopic pregnancy. In: Chamberlain G (ed) Contemporary gynaecology. Butterworths, London, p 57

Stabile I, Grudzinskas J G 1990 Ectopic pregnancy: a review of incidence, etiology and diagnostic aspects. Obstetrical and Gynaecological Survey 45: 375–347

Sutton C J S 1989 Laparoscopic surgery. Clinical Obstetrics and Gynaecology 3: 429–686

Turnbull A, Chamberlain G (eds) 1989 Obstetrics. Churchill Livingstone, Edinburgh

GESTATIONAL TROPHOBLASTIC DISEASE (GTD)

Hydatidiform mole (HM)

Incidence

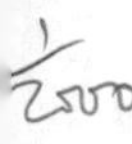

The worldwide range is 0.2 to 2.0 per 1000 pregnancies for population-based studies. For hospital-based studies it is 0.7 to 11.5 per 1000 births. The incidence in England and Wales, and in the USA, is about 1.5 per 1000 livebirths.

There are two types of hydatidiform mole:

1. *Complete mole (CHM)* — the conceptus consists solely of hyperplastic, hydropic chorionic villi; no fetus is present. It usually results from fertilisation of an ovum which then loses its nucleus. The haploid sperm duplicates its own chromosomes by meiosis. The result is that:
   (i) The chromosome complement is usually homozygous 46 XX derived solely from the father (androgenetic)
   (ii) Only one pair of paternal HLA antigens is expressed
   About 10% of CHM are heterozygous — usually 46XY but sometimes 46XX. They arise from fertilisation of an anucleate egg by two sperm. CHM uniquely combine paternal nuclear DNA with maternal mitochondrial DNA. Women with CHM have an increased incidence of balanced translocations and this could explain the loss of the ovum nucleus.
2. *Partial mole (PHM)* — there is focal hyperplasia of trophoblast with varying degrees of hydropic villous degeneration; a fetus is present. Chromosomal abnormalities (particularly triploidy-69, XXX or XXY) are often found. The source of the extra set of chromosomes may be double fertilisation (dispermy) or failure of the first paternal meiotic division

Risk markers for HM

1. *Age* — increased for CHM (but not PHM) at extremes of reproductive life (>30 years and <15 years of age)
2. *Ethnic group* — the traditionally reported excess in South-East Asia has decreased and may have been explained by reliance on hospital- rather than population-based data, and greater incidence of pregnancy in young and older women. In the USA, HM may be less frequent among black women compared with women of other racial groups
3. *Obstetric history*
   (i) *Previous HM*

Number of previous HM	Risk in next pregnancy
1	1:75
2*	1:65

*These women still have a 75% chance of a next successful pregnancy

4. (ii) *Previous multiple pregnancy* — twinning and HM may both represent different defects in gametogenesis or fertilisation

Symptoms

Most are related to excessive production of hCG.

1. Amenorrhoea combined with exaggerated pregnancy symptoms e.g. hyperemesis gravidarum
2. There may be irregular vaginal bleeding and the loss may contain the classical vesicles; many present as incomplete miscarriages
3. Pre-eclampsia may develop unusually early
4. Hyperthyroidism develops in about 5% of women with CHM
5. Massive trophoblastic embolisation may cause respiratory distress requiring prompt treatment (see Suggested further reading)

Signs

1. The uterus may be large for dates
2. Ovaries may be palpably enlarged due to presence of theca — lutein cysts

Diagnosis

1. B-hCG can be markedly raised in serum and urine, but most patients have values within the normal range for pregnancy
2. Ultrasound — the characteristic 'snow-storm' appearance is not pathognomonic. In CHM fetal parts are absent. PHM and missed abortion can be confused

Invasive mole (IM)

There is local invasion of the myometrium and it is therefore much less readily removed by evacuation. The tumour may perforate the uterus. Vaginal metastases may also occur but more distant spread is uncommon. This is a histological diagnosis usually made after hysterectomy which has become necessary because vaginal bleeding has continued and hCG levels have remained raised after initial attempts to empty the uterus. There is usually a good response to chemotherapy.

Placental site trophoblastic tumour (PSTT)
This is a rare form which appears to arise from placental bed trophoblast rather than the usual villous origin for HM etc. Most cases follow within 3 years of miscarriage or term pregnancy. It can be associated with hypertension and the nephrotic syndrome. The response to chemotherapy is poor, and hysterectomy is indicated (unless metastasis is advanced).

Gestational choriocarcinoma
This is a highly malignant tumour characterised by disordered growth of syncytio- and cytotrophoblast and invasion of the myometrium causing necrosis and haemorrhage. Metastasis is common. It usually arises within 2 years of the causal pregnancy.

Incidence
About 1 in 20 000 to 1 in 40 000 pregnancies in Western countries increasing to about 1 in 13 000 pregnancies in the Far East.

Risk markers for choriocarcinoma
1. Age — as for CHM
2. Obstetric history — only about 1 in 30 hydatidiform moles develop into choriocarcinoma. However, the risk of subsequent choriocarcinoma is 1000 times greater after a mole than after a normal pregnancy. Thus, as many cases follow moles as follow other pregnancies. Heterozygous CHM have a greater malignant potential than do homozygous CHM
3. ABO blood group — the risk of choriocarcinoma is increased when the woman and her partner have different ABO groups. Groups B and AB patients have a less good prognosis.
4. HLA compatibility between partners may be associated with increased risk of developing choriocarcinoma

Pathology
Local extension is frequent but ovarian spread is uncommon. The predominant route of spread is vascular. Lymphatic spread is rare. Pulmonary metastases occur in about 70% of cases. They may have a 'cannon-ball' or 'snow-storm' appearance or

appear intravascular on chest X-ray. Haemoptysis is a common symptom.

Staging of GTD

Stage 0	Molar pregnancy
Stage I	Persistently elevated hCG titres (i.e. 6 months or more after evacuation) and tumour confined to body of uterus
Stage II	Pelvic and/or vaginal metastasis
Stage III	Pulmonary metastasis
Stage IV	All other distant metastases

A prognostic scoring system can be used in Stages I to IV to determine the appropriate treatment for each patient. For details see Suggested further reading. It is based on:

1. The extent of the tumour burden, e.g. hCG level, and number, site and size of metastases
2. Patient characteristics, e.g. risk increases with age and parity
3. The nature of and the interval since the antecedent pregnancy:
   (i) The risk is highest for a term pregnancy and lowest for a hydatidiform mole
   (ii) The longer the interval the higher the risk
4. The patient's ability to respond immunologically, e.g.
   (i) A well-developed lymphocytic infiltrate around the tumour is a favourable feature
   (ii) ABO blood groups of both partners
5. Poor response to previous chemotherapy

Management of GTD

Stage 0

1. Once a firm diagnosis is made the mole needs to be removed preferably by suction evacuation and curettage. This may need to be repeated if: (a) irregular bleeding persists, or (b) hCG levels are still elevated 6 weeks after initial evacuation. Hysterectomy can be carried out in older women whose family is complete
2. In the UK, patients should be registered with one of the three reference laboratories
3. *Follow-up*
   (i) hCG estimations should be carried out on 24-hour urine samples weekly until levels are normal (<100 i.u. day), monthly for a year and then 3-monthly during the second year
   (ii) The patient may begin to try to become pregnant 6 months after hCG values have become and remain normal. A barrier method of contraception should be used until hCG levels are normal: then oral contraception can be used. There may be a higher

incidence of subsequent choriocarcinoma if the 'pill' is started before hCG levels fall. hCG levels should be checked 3 weeks after the end of any pregnancy subsequent to a molar pregnancy

4. Chemotherapy is not necessary unless the disease progresses. Among the signs of this are:
   (i) Urinary hCG levels > 40 000 i.u./day 6 weeks after evacuation
   (ii) Any elevation of hCG levels 6 months after evacuation
   (iii) Persistent or recurrent uterine bleeding with raised urinary hCG levels

Management of Stages I–IV should be confined to specialised centres (see Suggested further reading).

Results of therapy
Remission can be expected in all women adequately treated in Stages I to III and in up to 70% of women with Stage IV disease.

Subsequent pregnancies
A normal outcome can be expected. The incidence of congenital malformation is not increased in women who have received chemotherapy.

SUGGESTED FURTHER READING

Hammond C B 1988 Trophoblastic disease. Obstetric and Gynaecology Clinics of North America 15: 435–590

Newlands E S 1983 Treatment of trophoblastic disease. In: Studd J (ed) Progress in obstetrics and gynaecology. Churchill Livingstone, Edinburgh, Vol 3, p. 13.

Turnbull A, Chamberlain G (eds) 1989 Obstetrics. Churchill Livingstone, Edinburgh

Congenital abnormalities

Malformation — a primary error in normal development of an organ or tissue.
Disruption — a secondary malformation resulting from damage to a previously normal organ or tissue. About 15% of newborns have a single minor malformation.
Major congenital malformations constitute 10% of miscarriages, 3% of all deliveries, under 2% of live births, and about 30% of all stillbirths, neonatal deaths and infant deaths. The incidence is more than doubled in multiple pregnancy (especially in monozygotic twins). Perinatal mortality due to malformations is around 2.5/1000 births. Thirty per cent of all children born alive with major malformations die within 5 years.
The birth incidence of major malformations is:

CNS	10/1000 births
CVS	8/1000 births
Renal tract	4/1000 births
Limbs	2/1000 births
Others	6/1000 births
Total	30/1000 births

Aetiology
The most important causes of congenital defects and their approximate incidence are as follows:

Idiopathic	60%
Multifactorial	20%
Single-gene disorders	7 to 8%
Chromosomal	6%
Infections	2%
Maternal illness (e.g. epilepsy, diabetes, PKU)	3%
Drugs, radiation, alcohol	1 to 2%

Deformation — an alteration in shape or position due to inappropriate mechanical forces. The most significant are congenital dislocation of the hip (CDH) and talipes equinovarus. They can have intrinsic or extrinsic causes and can be associated with: neuromuscular or connective tissue disorders, and CNS malformation (intrinsic); or oligohydramnios, malpresentations, uterine anomalies and multiple pregnancy (extrinsic). About 2% of newborns are affected; one third of these have multiple deformations.

CYTOGENETICS

The normal human karyotype has 46 chromosomes: 22 pairs of autosomes, and 2 sex chromosomes — XX in the normal female and XY in the normal male.

Each chromosome has: a *centromere* — the narrow waist which may be near the middle (metacentric), close to one end (acrocentric), or in an intermediate position (submetacentric); a long arm (q) and a short arm (p); and a *telomere* at the tip of each arm.

Mitosis — a process by which all somatic cells divide. It involves splitting of each of the 46 chromosomes to provide a full identical (diploid) complement for both daughter cells. It is divided arbitrarily into five stages:

1. *Interphase* — the period between successive cell divisions
2. *Prophase* — the chromatids split longitudinally into pairs of chromatids connected at the centromere
3. *Metaphase* — movement of the chromatids occurs towards the equator of the cell
4. *Anaphase* — the centromeres divide, and the paired chromatids separate
5. *Telophase* — the cytoplasm divides, the chromosomes unwind, and two genetically identical daughter cells are formed

Meiosis — a process by which all germ cells (gametes) divide and during which the chromosome of the daughter cells is halved (haploid). Two sequential cell divisions are involved:

1. Interchange or cross-over of chromosomal material can take place during prophase of the first division; daughter cells inherit chromatid pairs still attached at the centromere
2. Completion of separation

Summary

The somatic cell produces by mitosis two diploid cells, each containing 46 chromosomes. The germ cell produces, by meiosis, four haploid gametes, each with 23 chromosomes. Gametogenesis is discussed on page 187.

CHROMOSOMAL DISORDERS

Ninety-five per cent of gametes with chromosome abnormalities are not viable. They affect at least 7% of all conceptions and 6 per 1000 of all livebirths. They are present in 60% of first-trimester miscarriages, 5% of second-trimester miscarriages, and 4 to 5% of stillbirths.

Abnormalities can be numerical or structural.

Numerical aberrations

1. *Aneuploidy* — an abnormality in number of chromosomes, usually by mutation. It can arise during meiosis or mitosis. It is usually due to the failure of paired chromosomes to separate at anaphase (non-disjunction), or their delayed movement at the same stage (anaphase lag). Two cells are produced, one with an extra copy of a chromosome (trisomy), the other with that chromosome missing (monosomy)
2. *Polyploidy* — the number of chromosomes is an exact multiple of the haploid, but greater than the diploid number, e.g. triploidy (69XXY is the most common), or tetraploidy (4n)

Structural aberrations

Due to chromosome breakage and inappropriate rejoining of the broken ends.

1. *Translocation* of fragments between chromosomes — often inherited:
   (i) A balanced translocation exists when the genome contains the correct amount of genetic matter and they usually have no outward manifestation. If one parent has a balanced translocation the theoretical outlook for any offspring is:
      1:4 have the same balanced translocation
      1:4 have normal chromosomes
      1:2 have an unbalanced translocation
   These rates are affected by a high spontaneous abortion rate
   (ii) Unbalanced translocations always declare themselves and occur when the genome contains extra genetic matter

   There are three types of translocation: (a) reciprocal, in which the chromosomal material distal to breaks in two chromosomes is exchanged; (b) Robertsonian, in which breaks in two acrocentric chromosomes (most commonly numbers 13 and 14) occur near the centromere with cross-fusion of the products; and (c) insertional, in which three breaks occur in one or two chromosomes
2. *Deletion* — loss of any part of a chromosome. Substantial losses are nearly always lethal. A *ring chromosome* can result if both arms of a chromosome break, the terminal ends are lost, and the two proximal sticky ends unite

3. *Duplication* — two copies of a chromosome segment are present. It is more common than deletion but generally less harmful
4. *Inversion* — two breaks occur in one chromosome with inversion of 180° of the segment between breaks. It does not usually produce a clinical abnormality but can give rise to unbalanced gametes.
5. *Isochromosome* — deletion of one and duplication of the other chromosome. The commonest in live births is that of the long arm of X which is a cause of Turner's syndrome (p. 32)

Other aberrations

1. *Mosaic* -- an individual with two or more cell lines derived from a single zygote
2. *Chimaera* — two cell lines are derived from two separate zygotes. It can arise by
   - (i) Early fusion of dizygotic twin zygotes
   - (ii) Double fertilisation of the egg and a polar body
   - (iii) Exchange of haemopoietic cells in utero between dizygotic twins

AUTOSOMAL ABNORMALITIES

Down syndrome

The overall incidence is 1:650 live births, and, although up to 50% of all affected conceptuses miscarry early, over one-third survive to viability.

Genetic abnormalities in Down syndrome

Trisomy 21 (due to non-disjunction)	95% (maternal age-related)
Translocation 14:21	2%
Other translocations	2%
Mosaicism	1%

Maternal age-related risk of trisomy 21

Maternal age (years)	*Approximate risk of affected child per 1000 live births*
20	1 in 2000
30	1 in 900
35	1 in 365
36	1 in 240
38	1 in 180
40	1 in 110
42	1 in 70
44	1 in 40
46	1 in 25
48	1 in 15

The risk of recurrence of Down syndrome due to trisomy 21 is about 1 in 100. For mothers aged 35 years or over, the risk of the Down syndrome or another chromosomal abnormality recurring is approximately four times the age-related risk.

The risk of translocation 14:21 recurring is about 1 in 10 if the mother has a balanced translocation; 1 in 50 if the father has it.

Prenatal diagnosis is discussed on p. 38.

Affected children have a characteristic 'mongoloid' facial appearance, and are mentally retarded to a varying degree. They are often happy and affectionate. Congenital heart disease may be present, and they are at increased risk of, for example, recurrent infections and acute leukaemia.

Other autosomal trisomies (13, 18 and 22)
Also maternal age-related: due to non-disjunction. Rare as livebirths. Recurrence risk is probably low.

SEX CHROMOSOME DISORDERS

Defect	*Incidence compared with live births*	*Average IQ*	*Association with maternal age*
XO	1:3000 (1:100 conceptions)	100	Incidence falls as age rises
XXX	1:1000	Possible slight reduction	Increased × 2–3 when maternal age > 40
XXY	1:700	100	Increased × 2–3 when maternal age > 40
XYY	1:700	100	None

These conditions have a much better outlook than was originally thought (for further discussion see p. 238–240). Antenatal detection does not necessarily warrant termination of pregnancy. About 5% XO females will have periods and a few may be fertile.

SINGLE GENE DISORDERS

1. Autosomal dominant conditions
These are often mild (e.g. polydactyly), have various degrees of manifestation or, if severe, arise during adulthood (e.g. renal polycystic disease) or at the end of the reproductive period (e.g. Huntington's chorea).

(i) The combined incidence of all dominants is 7/1000 live births
(ii) Fifty per cent of the offspring of an affected individual will be affected. The commonest dominant condition is familial hypercholesterolaemia (up to 4/1000 of the population)

Among others, less frequent, are:

Huntington's chorea	Ehler–Danlos syndrome
Neurofibromatosis	Spherocytosis
Tuberous sclerosis	Otosclerosis
Achondroplasia	Polyposis coli
Marfan's syndrome	Adult polycystic disease of the kidneys

Advanced ultrasound techniques, cordocentesis and molecular genetics are making the diagnosis of an increasing number of these conditions possible (see p. 40).

2. Autosomal recessive conditions

The gene must be inherited from both parents. The effects are usually severe. Fifty per cent of offspring of affected individuals will be carriers.

There are racial differences in the frequency of some of these conditions. Among those with the highest overall incidence are shown in the following table.

Approximate incidence in different populations (per 1000 births)

Cystic fibrosis	North Europeans (0.4–0.5)	Negroes/orientals (0.001)
Thalassaemias	Mediterranean people/orientals (up to 20)	North Europeans (Insignificant)
Sickle-cell anaemia	Negroes (up to 20)	North Europeans (Insignificant)
Tay–Sachs disease	Ashkenazi Jews (up to 0.4)	Sephardi Jews/gentiles (Insignificant)
Severe autosomal recessive mental retardation	UK incidence 0.5	
Phenylketonuria	UK incidence about 0.1 (higher in north-west than south-east)	
Many other inborn errors of metabolism	Too many for overall incidence to be meaningful	

Prediction of risk or detection of the conditions is based on:

(i) Screening high risk populations for heterozygote carriers before pregnancy or marriage. There are serious social and ethical difficulties in this approach (loss of marital freedom, social stigma, etc.). It has been useful among American Jews for Tay–Sachs disease but less so for sickle-cell disease and thalassaemia in high-risk groups

(ii) Chorionic villus biopsy or amniocentesis in early pregnancy after previous affected child, e.g. for inborn errors of metabolism

(iii) Cordocentesis after previous affected child or when parents are known to be heterozygote carriers, e.g. thalassaemias, sickle cell disease. Prenatal diagnosis is considered more fully on pp. 38–44

(iv) Neonatal screening (see p. 160 for phenylketonuria)

Thalassaemias

Autosomal recessively inherited defects in the rate of synthesis of one or more globin chains:

(i) Alpha-thalassaemia is due to the deletion of structural DNA genes affecting the alpha-Hb chains

(ii) HbF contains alpha chains, therefore the fetus can be affected to an extent varying from anaemia to hydrops

(iii) Beta-thalassaemia is due to a messenger RNA abnormality causing defective production of β-Hb chains:
β^+ disease — reduced production of β chains
β° disease — no β chains
In β° and β^+ disease homozygotes are affected severely, (thalassaemia major) from which up to 100 000 children die world-wide each year

Sickle-cell disease

This is due to structural alterations in one of the globin chains. There are more than 80 alpha chains and 180 beta chain variants; the most important clinically are HbS and HbC. HbS/S is commonest and most troublesome in tropical Africa (heterozygote frequency 20–40%). It is also present among North American blacks (heterozygote frequency 9%), in the Middle East, India and the Mediterranean littoral. HbS/C affects West Indian Negro populations particularly severely.

The high world-wide frequency of the sickle-cell and thalassaemia genes probably occurs because heterozygotes are protected against falciparum malaria.

Phenylketonuria (PKU)

Locus found on chromosome 12. Carrier detection and prenatal diagnosis in affected families is now possible using DNA analysis (see p. 43). Routine neonatal screening is still mandatory.

A mother with PKU has about an 8% chance of having an affected child. She must receive a phenylalanine-free diet from *before* conception, otherwise the risk of spontaneous abortion, infant death or severe mental retardation is high, even if the child has not inherited the disorder.

Cystic fibrosis (CF)

This is the commonest inherited metabolic disorder in Western populations. Its UK incidence is about 1 in 1600 births and the carrier frequency is about 1 in 22.

The cystic fibrosis gene has been found on chromosome 7.

The commonest mutation causing CF accounts for only up to 70% of cases, and another 10 to 12 mutations account for the rest. Carrier detection for the commonest mutation is possible, but 30% of carriers will not be detected. Currently it should be offered to members of cystic fibrosis families and their partners. Rapid advances in this field are likely.

Women with CF are now living longer, and a few pregnancies have been reported. The risk of pre-term delivery and maternal and perinatal mortality seem to be increased. Women with severe respiratory impairment should be strongly advised to avoid pregnancy.

Infantile polycystic disease
Results in cysts in the kidneys, liver and pancreas which are usually lethal. Prenatal screening is possible using serial ultrasound examination of the fetal kidneys.

3. X-Linked disorders
X-linked disorders are recessive and cause concern in families known to be affected. Among the disorders are:

Duchenne's muscular dystrophy — 0.3/1000 males
Fragile X-associated mental retardation — 0.5/1000 males
Haemophilia A — factor VIII deficiency — 0.2/1000 males
Haemophilia B — factor IX deficiency — 0.03/1000 males
Red/green colour blindness — 80/1000 males

All the daughters of affected males are carriers but none of their sons will be affected. Thus a woman is a heterozygote if she has:

(i) an affected father
(ii) two affected sons
(iii) an affected brother with an affected son
(iv) an affected daughter with an affected son
(v) two daughters both with affected sons

In addition, heterozygosity can be suspected in the presence of slight abnormalities in the appropriate biochemistry (e.g. factors VIII and IX) but there is an overlap with the normal range.

Antenatal detection of fetuses with Duchenne's muscular dystrophy, fragile X or haemophilia is now possible using DNA analysis (see p. 43).

MULTIFACTORIAL DISORDERS

The most significant conditions within this group are neural tube defects, many congenital heart lesions, facial clefts, diaphragmatic herniae, and gut atresias.

Neural tube defects (NTD)
Anencephaly and spina bifida comprise 95% of NTDs and encephalocoele the remaining 5%. The incidence:

1. Shows marked geographical variation
   USA, Canada, Japan, Africa — 1 per 1000 births
   SE England — 3 per 1000 births
   W Scotland — 5 per 1000 births
   S Wales — 7 to 8 per 1000 births
   N Ireland — 8 to 9 per 1000 births
   Eire — 10 per 1000 births
   It occurs more frequently in winter births. In the UK the recurrence risk after one affected child is 1 in 25, rising to 1 in 10 after two or more. An affected parent has a 1 in 25 risk of producing a child with a NTD.
2. Is inversely related to socio-economic status
3. Has dropped steadily over the past 20 years — this is not entirely accounted for by antenatal screening programmes

Prevention of NTD

The risk of recurrence may be reduced if multivitamin tablets, which include folic acid, are taken from at least 1 month before conception to about 8 weeks of pregnancy.

Congenital heart lesions

The overall incidence has inexplicably increased over the past 15 years and is now 8 per 1000 births.

The incidence and recurrence risks for various types of congenital heart defects are given in the following table.

	Birth incidence	*Recurrence risks*	
		Sibs	*Offspring*
Ventricular septal defect	1 in 400	1 in 25	
Atrial septal defect	1 in 1000	1 in 33	
Tetralogy of Fallot	1 in 1000	1 in 33:	1 in 25
Coarctation of aorta	1 in 1600	1 in 50	
Aortic stenosis	1 in 2000	1 in 50:	1 in 33
Transposition of the great vessels	1 in 16 000	1 in 50:	unknown

Prenatal diagnosis of some of the most serious of the defects is possible using high-resolution ultrasound imaging and fetal echocardiography at 18 to 20 weeks (see p. 41).

Facial clefts

Cleft lip and/or palate occurs in 1 per 1000 births. Most are multifactorial but it is associated with over 150 rare single-gene traits or chromosomal abnormalities (e.g. trisomy 13). Surgical repair with good results is usual. Recurrence risks for the multifactorial lesions are:

1. Child with unilateral cleft lip in normal parents: 1 in 50
2. Child with bilateral cleft lips and palate in normal parents: 1 in 20

Isolated cleft palate is distinct. It affects 1 in 2500 births, with a recurrence risk of 1 in 50 for sibs and offspring.

Anterior abdominal wall defects
These occur in about 1 in 6000 pregnancies, and the two main forms are:

1. *Exomphalos* — the umbilical cord is involved and is attached to the apex of the sac which may contain liver and/or intestines. Associated chromosomal anomalies occur in 30% and cardiac lesions in 10%
2. *Gastroschisis* — the umbilical cord is not involved and there is no sac. Associated gut atresias and cardiac lesions (but not chromosome abnormalities) occur in up to 20%.
   Prenatal diagnosis by ultrasound is possible. Maternal serum AFP may be elevated. Chromosomal anomalies should be excluded if exomphalos is suspected. Vaginal delivery should be aimed for except for obstetric indications. Isolated defects are often correctable surgically
3. *Body stalk anomalies* form a third, less common defect. They are associated with major lower body deformities

Gastrointestinal anomalies
Among those with multifactorial inheritance patterns are:

1. *Hirschsprung disease* — 1 in 8000 newborn affected with a 3-to-1 male excess.

	Recurrence risk	
	Sibs	Offspring
Affected male	1 in 25:	<1 in 100
Affected female	1 in 8:	<1 in 100

2. *Pyloric stenosis* — incidence in males is 1 in 200; in females it is 1 in 1000. The greatest risk of recurrence is in male relatives of a female patient (1 in 6). The lowest risk is for female relatives of a male patient (1 in 50). The risks for the other two possible combinations are intermediate
3. *Oesophageal atresia/tracheo-oesophageal fistula* — affect 1 in 3000 newborns. May be associated with cardiac defects. Can be suspected prenatally by persistent absence of stomach bubble on ultrasound
4. *Gut atresias* — may occur at any level of the intestine and affect 1 in 330 newborns. Can be diagnosed prenatally by ultrasound
5. *Diaphragmatic hernia* — occurs in between 1 in 2000 and 1 in 5000 births: 95% of affected fetuses are stillborn. The incidence of associated anomalies may be as high as 60% overall

Other malformations
Obstructive uropathies. Dilatation of whole or part of urinary tract most commonly due to urethral valves. Affects males 20 times more often than females. The prognosis depends on the time of onset and severity of the obstruction. The dilated urinary tract can be observed ultrasonically in the fetus. The role of fetal therapy is discussed on p. 43.

GENETIC COUNSELLING AND PRENATAL DIAGNOSIS

Ethical issues — knowledge about and techniques for studying fetal development in general and genetics in particular are advancing rapidly. This increases our responsibility to consider the ethical issues raised. 'What *can* we do?' must be balanced by 'What *ought* we to do?'. Among the ethical dilemmas we face are:

1. General population screening for defective genes, e.g. the cystic fibrosis gene
2. Testing of pre-implantation embryos after assisted conception
3. More aggressive prenatal screening for conditions causing varying degrees of disability, e.g. Down's syndrome
4. False-positive rates inherent in all screening programmes

Genetic counselling is the imparting of knowledge and advice about inherited conditions. This involves:

1. Complete history from or about the affected individual (proband)
2. Construction of pedigree
3. Physical examination of proband with particular reference to dysmorphic features
4. Accurate diagnosis — among the indications for chromosome analysis are:
   Family history of chromosomal aberration
   Dysmorphic features
   Multiple congenital anomalies
   Ambiguous genitalia
   Unexplained short stature in female
   Unexplained mental retardation
   Unexplained stillbirth
   Recurrent miscarriage (see p. 16)
   Some forms of cancer associated with chromosomal rearrangements, e.g. neuroblastoma, leukaemia, retinoblastoma, Wilm's tumour
5. Non-directive counselling — see Connor and Ferguson-Smith in Suggested further reading
6. Follow-up

Prenatal diagnosis can be justified if the condition

1. Is severe in its effects

2. Has a high genetic risk
3. Is untreatable

The test must be reliable, and must be preceded by counselling. Tests for those anomalies which can be diagnosed antenatally can be applied:

1. As a *screening test* in a whole population to define a subgroup at particular risk with whom diagnostic procedures can be discussed. The best example of this is serum AFP screening for NTD
2. As *diagnostic tests* in a group of women at high risk of a particular problem, e.g. older mothers and Down syndrome: a previous personal or family history of chromosomal disorders or inborn errors of metabolism: women with 'positive' screening tests

The basis of diagnosis is either:

1. The search for characteristic intracellular defects in fetal tissue obtained by invasive procedures (see below), or
2. The visualisation of morphological defects by ultrasound

Antenatal screening for NTD using alpha-feto protein (AFP)
The aim is to identify a population of women at high enough risk to justify diagnostic procedures. Policies for and against screening must be determined by the prevalence of the condition within each district or region. The balance between risk and benefit must consider that the screening procedure can provoke anxiety amongst unaffected women.

A cut-off level for serum AFP of around 2.5 multiples of the normal median (MoM) at 16–18 weeks' gestation will detect 90% of anencephaly, 80% of open spina bifida, but will include 3% of unaffected singleton pregnancies.

Each laboratory must work out the 'cut-off' levels best suited to its circumstances.

High-quality ultrasound examination is vital to check gestational age, seek for a cranial or spinal defect, and exclude multiple pregnancy, intrauterine death or other associated conditions (see below). Routine ultrasound is increasingly being used for screening for NTD and other anomalies (see below), and a 'normal' detailed ultrasonic examination may reassure the mother without amniocentesis being necessary. If amniocentesis is carried out, amniotic fluid levels of AFP greater than 5 standard deviations above the mean suggest the possibility of NTD. Detailed ultrasound and the discovery of an abnormal band of acetylcholinesterase on electrophoresis in affected cases both help to clarify the diagnosis.

AFP and other fetal problems
High serum and amniotic fluid AFP levels may be associated with conditions such as exomphalos, congenital nephrosis,

posterior urethral valves, Turner's syndrome and trisomy 13. High serum AFP alone predicts an increased risk of a variety of obstetric problems, including IUGR and perinatal death, particularly if oligohydramnios is present.

Clinical procedures

Biochemical screening for Down syndrome
Even if all pregnant women aged 35 years or over elected to have an amniocentesis, this would result in a detection rate for Down syndrome of 35% for an amniocentesis rate of 7.5%. Increased detection rates may be achievable by measuring AFP, unconjugated oestriol (E_3), and hCG at 16–18 weeks and calculating a maternal age specific related risk of Down syndrome. AFP and E_3 tend to be reduced and hCG increased in affected pregnancies. At a risk cut-off level of 1 in 200, biochemical screening could raise the detection level to 60% with an amniocentesis rate of 5%. This policy would carry a 4% false-positive rate. It has not yet been prospectively tested.

In some cases ultrasound examination may raise the index of suspicion.

1. Ultrasonography
This has become the main diagnostic technique for prenatal diagnosis of congenital anomalies by allowing:

1. Direct visualisation of the defect, e.g. anencephaly
2. Detection of markers of chromosomal defects
3. Accurate direction of instruments during invasive diagnostic (or therapeutic) procedures

It can be achieved as part of a policy for routine examination at 16 to 20 weeks, or in women at greater than average risk of particular disorders. Detailed ultrasound requires great interpretative skill from the operator if unacceptable levels of false-positive and false-negative diagnosis are to be avoided. Some of the more sophisticated techniques should be carried out in regional centres with the appropriate expertise. The following table highlights some specific points. For more detailed discussion see Suggested further reading.

Condition	*Ultrasonic examination*	*Comment*
Spina bifida	(i) BPD and head circumference reduced; (ii) ventriculomegaly; (iii) scalloping of frontal bones ('lemon sign'); (iv) anterior curve of cerebellar hemispheres ('banana sign') or absent	Reliable when examined by experienced personnel. The presence of some of these signs indicates need for more detailed examination

Condition	Ultrasonic examination	Comment
	cerebellum (all at 16–18 weeks)	
Congenital heart defects	'Four chamber' view of heart at transverse section of thorax	Optimum time for examination: 18 to 24 weeks
	Echocardiography for individual women at high risk	For specialised centres only
Down syndrome	Ratio of bi-parietal to occipito-frontal diameter to detect brachycephaly	Of no value in population screening
	Nuchal skin thickness	(i) May occur in normal fetuses; (ii) varies with attitude of fetal head; (iii) can be produced artificially by angle of transducer
	Short femur (using increased BPD:femur length ratio as index)	May be useful as ancillary screening method at 16 weeks

Fetal blood sampling by cordocentesis under ultrasonic guidance has replaced fetoscopy as the method of choice. Its primary diagnostic applications are:

1. Haemoglobinopathies, Von Willebrand's disease
2. X-linked disorders, e.g. haemophilia A and B; Duchenne muscular dystrophy if fetus found to be male by CV biopsy in women at risk
3. Exclusion of fetal injection — particularly rubella. Fetal blood sampling is best performed at about 18 weeks' gestation; the sample is taken from the area of the insertion of the cord into the placenta

Anti-D immunoglobulin (100 μg, or more if Kleihauer indicates it) should be given to Rh-D-negative women carrying Rh-D-positive fetuses.

The risk of fetal loss is probably between 1 and 2% in expert hands. Its use should be confined to centres with such expertise.

2. Chorionic villus (CV) biopsy

CV biopsy obtains fetal tissue from the chorion at the edge of the placenta under ultrasound guidance. One technique uses a transcervical approach between 8 and 12 weeks. The second, and now more popular, transabdominal route can be used from 8 weeks to term. The additional procedure-related risk of miscarriage is about 2%. Its potential advantages are:

(i) It can be carried out in the first trimester
(ii) The tissue is ideal for DNA analysis and gene probing (see below)
(iii) Initial chromosome analysis can be ready in about 48 hours (full cultures still take 2–3 weeks)

However, the genetic composition of the chorion (trophoblast) is not necessarily the same as that of the fetus. For example, mosaicism and some rare trisomies confined to the trophoblast are not uncommon. Chromosomal aberrations found after CV biopsy must therefore be assessed carefully and with advice from a clinical geneticist.

3. Amniocentesis

This is usually carried out between 16 and 18 weeks' gestation but earlier testing is now being achieved. Earlier diagnosis would be a benefit, but complications and culture failure may be more common.

Indications:

1. Maternal age 38 or over
2. A screening test suggests high risk of serious disorder
3. Previous infant affected by a condition diagnosable antenatally
4. Family or personal history of diagnosable condition.

Risks:

1. Miscarriage — the excess procedure-related risk is between 0.5 and 1%. It is related to experience and use of ultrasound guidance. It is also increased when maternal serum AFP is elevated before testing
2. Postural deformities — e.g. talipes. This is questionable but may relate to the volume of liquor removed
3. Respiratory difficulties in newborn which remain unexplained

Precautions:

1. Always use ultrasound to localise the placenta and locate the liquor pool
2. Take sequestrene blood sample 20 minutes after the test to check for feto-maternal transfusion (Kleihauer test) in Rh-D-negative women
3. Give anti-D immunoglobulin 50 μg in all antibody-negative, Rh-D-negative women and to those whose Rh group is unknown. More can be given to cover any serious feto-maternal transfusion (see p. 88)

4. Fetoscopy

This is a highly specialised technique, the indications for which have decreased with advances in ultrasound. The main indication is for fetal biopsy — e.g. skin, muscle or liver. The risk of miscarriage due to fetoscopy is about 10%.

5. Embryo biopsy
IVF and embryo culture allow sampling of one or two cells at 8- to 16-cell stage.
DNA analysis of a single cell and/or karyotyping of cultured cell could be used for diagnosis of genetic defect in women at high risk of a serious disorder.
Only normal embryos would be reimplanted.
This is potentially more acceptable than later prenatal diagnostic methods.
It could ultimately allow 'gene therapy' in some cases.
However, even if the embryos are 'normal' the rate of successful pregnancies will be reduced.

Laboratory techniques
It is in this area that the most rapid advances are being made, particularly in molecular genetics (see Suggested further reading). Fetal cells can be analysed for:
1. Autosomal and sex chromosome anomalies (p. 32)
2. Enzyme production — over 80 inborn errors of metabolism are amenable to prenatal diagnosis
3. DNA analysis:
   (i) Using gene- or chromosome-region-specific probes — the presence or absence of the gene associated with the condition can be confirmed
   (ii) DNA amplification by the *polymerase chain reaction*. The relevant DNA fragment can be identified on an electrophoretic gel. This technique has many practical clinical genetic applications
   (iii) *Pulsed-field gel electrophoresis* allows separation of large fragments of DNA. It is useful for identifying gene deletion causing genetic disorders

FETAL THERAPY

1. Medical
Intravascular infusions or injections are possible by cordocentesis under ultrasound control. For example:
1. Transfusion to correct anaemia secondary to Rh iso-immunisation
2. Protein infusion to correct hypoproteinaemia due to non-immune hydrops
3. Platelet infusion or immunoglobulin (Ig) injection for allo-immune thrombocytopaenia (see p. 86)
4. Direct injection to treat fetal hypothyroidism or cardiac failure

2. Surgical
Ultrasound-guided techniques can be used to:
1. Drain pleural effusions or ascites

2. Insert ventriculo-amniotic shunts to reduce hydrocephalus. The results are bad, and this is not advised
3. Insert vesico-amniotic shunts to relieve obstructive uropathies. No consensus exists about criteria for this. In selected cases decompression may restore amniotic fluid volume and prevent pulmonary hypoplasia. It is unlikely to prevent or reverse renal damage

Fetal karyotypes should be obtained before any intervention is carried out.

Extrauterine surgery for fetal diaphragmatic hernia, obstructive uropathies, or even some cardiac defects has been attempted by hysterotomy, with the fetus returned to the uterus postoperatively. This is experimental and unlikely to have any place in clinical practice.

Post-mortem examination of fetuses

An experienced perinatal pathologist should be asked to examine all mid-trimester spontaneous abortions and those induced because of suspected congenital malformations. This will allow: (i) accurate counselling of the families, and (ii) audit of the screening and diagnostic tests. This is discussed further under Perinatal Mortality.

SUGGESTED FURTHER READING

Connor J M, Ferguson-Smith M A 1987 Essential medical genetics. 2nd edn. Blackwell Scientific Publications, Oxford

Dewhurst J, de Swiet M, Chamberlain G V P 1986 Basic science in obstetrics and gynaecology. Churchill Livingstone, Edinburgh

Harper P S 1984 Practical genetic counselling. 2nd edn. Wright, Bristol

Turnbull A, Chamberlain G (eds) 1989 Obstetrics. Churchill Livingstone, Edinburgh

Assessment of fetal growth and well-being

NORMAL FETAL GROWTH

Fetal growth and fetal size are often confused in clinical practice (see below). The average weights of normal fetuses as pregnancy progresses are:

Gestational age (weeks)	10	20	30	40
Approximate weight (g)	5	300	1500	3400

About 95% of birthweights fall within a normal distribution curve but the remaining 5% show a prolonged tail of low birthweight which is discussed below.

Factors affecting fetal growth and size

1. Physiological

1. *Genetic control*. This predominates in the first half of pregnancy, but environmental factors and other constraints give rise to greater variability in the second half of pregnancy. About 15% of total birthweight variation is attributable to the fetal genotype
2. *Fetal sex*. On average males weigh 150–200 g more than females at term. There is no difference up to 33 weeks' gestation
3. *Race*. The approximate mean birthweight for six ethnic groups are as follows:

Europeans	3200 g	Indonesians and Africans	3000 g
East and South-west Asians	3100 g	Indians	2900 g

   These differences do not solely depend on race; nutritional and socio-economic factors are likely to be involved
4. *Parental height and weight*. The paternal contribution is solely genetic. Maternal height and weight have independent effects on birthweight. Tall, heavy mothers will have babies up to 500 g heavier than short, light mothers
5. *Maternal age*. Teenage mothers and those over 35 years of age tend to have smaller babies (as well as an increased

incidence of congenital anomaly). Socio-economic factors also play a role
6. *Birth order.* Birthweight rises from first to second pregnancies by about 130 g, with a smaller rise in the third pregnancy. This may be associated with increased maternal weight
7. *Multiple pregnancy.* Twin growth is similar to singletons up to 32 weeks but decreases therafter. Dizygotic twins tend to be heavier than monozygotic. No weight-for-gestation standards exist for multiple pregnancy

2. Socio-economic
The average birthweight of babies born into social classes I and II (professional and managerial) is 150 g greater than for babies born into social classes IV and V. This may be related to maternal size, age and smoking habits rather than to nutritional status. In general, the growing fetus is protected against the effects of maternal deprivation unless they are very severe

3. Pathological markers for reduced fetal growth
1. *Previous obstetric history.* Women whose first pregnancy ended in stillbirth (but not miscarriage), or in birth of a growth-retarded baby, tend to have relatively small babies in subsequent pregnancies
2. *Smoking and altitude.* Smoking in pregnancy reduces the mean birthweight by 100 to 200 g from 34 weeks' gestation onwards. Nicotine and carbon monoxide pass through the placenta readily. Birthweight falls by about 100 g for every 1000 metres of altitude
3. Excessive alcohol ingestion (see p. 55)
4. Hypertensive syndromes (particularly pre-eclampsia)
5. Congenital malformation of fetus
6. Fetal or maternal infections
7. Multiple pregnancy

Weight-for-gestation standards
Weight-for-gestation standards are statistical reference levels which enable babies from similar populations to be defined and compared in a uniform manner in terms of weight and gestational age. Standard percentile values for birthweight can be found in Suggested further reading but need to be established for each population. They are usually derived from cross-sectional studies and reflect fetal size but *not* fetal growth (see below). The common standard selects a higher proportion of female than male infants from first rather than subsequent pregnancies because the average female infant is lighter than the average male, and because first babies tend to be lighter than subsequent ones. Corrections are therefore made for

gestational age and sex, and can also be made for birth order. There may have been a decline in mean birthweight-for-gestation between 1950 and 1980 despite social improvements and medical advances. Later data are not available.

Clinical use of weight-for-gestation standards
Size (as assessed by weight) at birth is important because, when the prognosis for an infant is dependent on the two variables, birthweight and gestational age, birthweight proves to be the more important. Most of the infants in whom problems will arise are found in the group found weighing less than the tenth percentile for gestational age and sex. These infants are termed 'small-for-dates' (SFD), 'light-for-dates' (LFD), 'small-for-gestational-age' (SGA), or 'light-for-gestational-age' (LGA). The last (LGA) is the most accurate description, though the first (SFD) is used commonly. The average birthweight of children with neurodevelopmental disability is significantly lower than it is for normal children.

Criticisms of weight-for-gestation standards
1. Cross-sectional data obtained at birth cannot be assumed to reflect longitudinal fetal growth
2. The weight of babies born at a given gestational age may not be representative of the babies at the same gestational age who remain *in utero*
3. Prediction of risk of death based on weight-for-gestational age centiles is relatively poor compared with prediction based on birthweight or gestational age alone
4. The charts do not identify those babies who are growth retarded but whose birthweight falls above the 10th centile
5. The charts do not correctly classify those babies who are normally grown but whose weight is below the tenth centile for gestational age and sex

Despite these criticisms, but as long as they are remembered, the tenth percentile cut-off for gestational age and sex for defining LGA infants is useful in clinical practice. Lowering the percentiles to the fifth or the third is useful in clinical research.

ASSESSMENT OF FETAL STATE

Fetal growth
1. Knowledge of gestational age. Menstrual history is an unreliable guide to gestational age in up to 45% of women. Uncertainty on the part of the women themselves is related to adverse outcomes such as perinatal death, low birthweight and spontaneous pre-term delivery independent of unfavourable maternal characteristics
2. More than one (and preferably serial) assessment of fetal size at least 2 weeks apart

Methods of assessment of gestational age and/or fetal growth

1. *Height of uterine fundus*. Clinical judgement of fundal height is not an accurate measure of gestational age, but it gives a guide to fetal growth. It is best measured as height (cm) above symphysis pubis as shown in the table below.

Gestational age (weeks)	*Average height (cm)*	*+ 2SDS*
20–31	Height = weeks	± 3
32–36	Height = (weeks − 1)	± 3
37–38	Height = (weeks − 2)	± 3
39–40	Height = (weeks − 3)	± 3

   Deviations from the above suggest the need for more detailed assessment, but the false-positive and false-negative rates are high
2. *Ultrasound — crown–rump (C–R) length*. At 7 weeks menstrual age the C–R length is 10 mm. This has increased to 55 mm by 12 weeks. It provides an accurate estimate of gestational age up to 14 weeks.
3. *Ultrasound-bi-parietal diameter (BPD)*. Serial measurements are widely used to measure fetal growth. When used to indicate fetal maturity it is most accurate before 24 weeks, but unreliable after 28 weeks
4. *Ultrasound — head/abdomen ratio*. Serial ultrasonic measurement of the ratio of the head circumference (at the level of the third ventricle) and the abdominal circumference (at the level of the umbilical vein) is a useful measure of fetal size and growth. It is especially useful in suspected intrauterine growth retardation (IUGR) when sparing of head growth makes BPD measurement less reliable. The ratio is therefore increased
5. *Ultrasound — femur length (FL)*. FL may be a more precise guide to gestational age than is BPD. Combining FL and BPD in a predictive formula (see Yagel in Suggested further reading) provides an accurate index of gestational age to 32 weeks

FETAL WELL-BEING

1. Fetal movements

A daily count of perceived fetal movements from 28 weeks' gestation is a simple and inexpensive routine screening device for monitoring fetal well-being. This can be done informally or formally using a 'kick-chart' in which mothers are asked to count the number of discrete fetal movements beginning at 9 a.m. each day. The time at which the tenth movement is felt is marked on the chart provided. Advice should be sought if fewer than 10 movements are perceived within 12 hours or if the mother feels that 'the baby is not moving'. Other tests of fetal welfare can then be applied.

Criticisms of fetal movement counts

1. Women may not perceive a large number of fetal movements
2. There are great variations in the number of fetal movements from day to day in individual women and from woman to woman
3. The sensitivity and specificity of the method is low
4. One randomised trial suggests a clear benefit, but another does not
5. Less than 1 per 1000 women might benefit from formal fetal movement counting using late fetal death as an outcome
6. Formal counting provokes anxiety in about 25% of women. Another 50% are reassured by it

2. Biochemical methods

1. *Indirect assessment*. The measurement of products of placental synthesis, such as *oestrogens* in maternal urine or plasma, and *human placental lactogen* in plasma, have faded from clinical practice; partly due to expense and poor predictive value for adverse outcomes, this is also a result of changes in fashion. Elevated levels of *maternal serum AFP* at 16 to 18 weeks' gestation in the absence of NTD predict some increased risk of growth retardation and other complications of pregnancy. The predictive value is not high but it can be used as a risk marker in determining patterns of antenatal care
2. *Direct fetal assessment*. It is possible to assess a variety of biochemical variables, e.g. hypoxia, acidaemia, hypoglycaemia by fetal blood sampling using cordocentesis under ultrasound control. If this is indicated at all it can only be in cases of severe fetal compromise

3. Antenatal fetal heart rate recording

The 'non-stress test' (NST) is widely used in the UK as a test of fetal welfare. The suggested programme is shown in the diagram on p. 50.

Contractions stress testing (CST) has been more popular in the USA. Contractions can be induced by an oxytocin infusion, or nipple stimulation. CST carries no benefits, and may have disadvantages over NST.

Interpretation of antenatal FHR recordings

Alterations in pattern are more subtle antenatally than intrapartum and the criteria for normality are not identical.

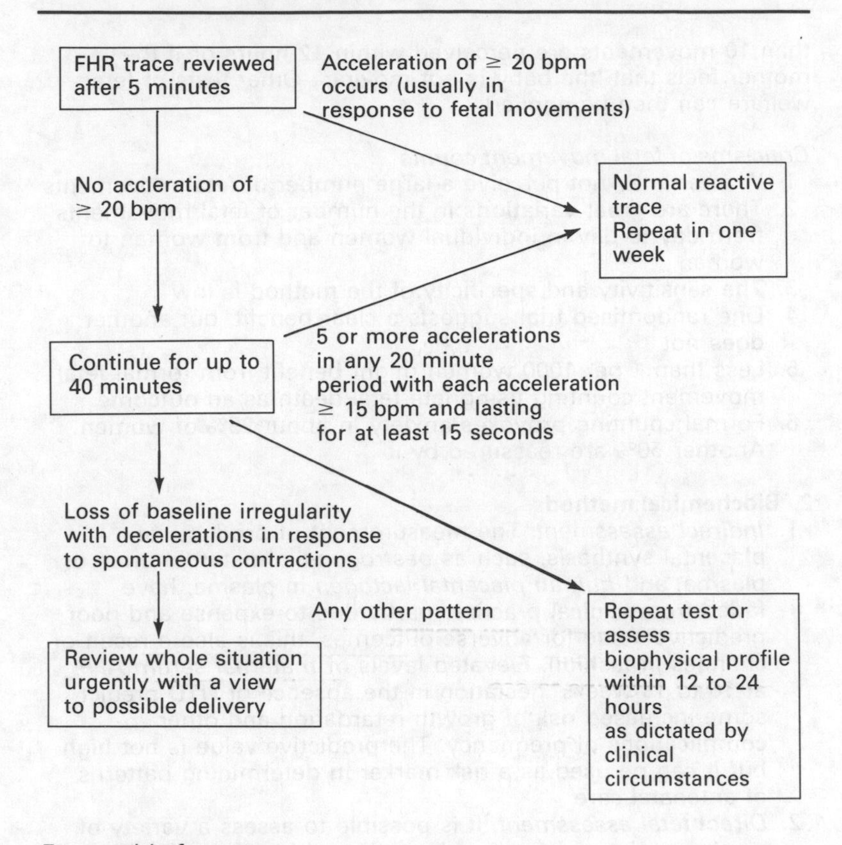

Favourable features:

1. Baseline irregularity > 10 bpm
2. Reactive patterns of FHR (i.e. acceleration with fetal movements)
3. No late decelerations with contractions

Unfavourable features:

1. Reduced or no baseline irregularity
2. Non-reactive patterns of FHR
3. Repeated late decelerations with contractions

Suspicious features:

1. Intermittent late decelerations
2. Persistent bradycardia or tachycardia
3. Variable decelerations
4. Poor-quality tracing or uterine hypertonus

The important feature which suggests that the fetus is in good health is the presence of discrete accelerations in response to fetal movements (a 'reactive trace'). Failure to show reactivity early in the trace is not necessarily abnormal because the fetus has 'rest–activity' cycles and the mean period of rest is about 40 minutes.

Baseline irregularity is an important feature. However, the earlier the gestation the more unreactive the normal trace is. The time from 28 to 32 weeks is a transitional period for the development of baseline irregularity.

Decelerations in relation to contractions accompanied by loss of baseline irregularity are a serious prognostic sign.

Criticisms of antenatal FHR

1. Visual assessments are liable to bias
2. Basal conditions are necessary for consistency
3. Trials of NST to screen for fetal compromise have not shown any benefit
4. They may be of value in women at higher risk of adverse outcome, but even this is not certain
5. The major hazards are over-interpretation and unnecessary intervention
6. Normal results are reassuring

4. Biophysical profile (BPP) scoring

BPP uses a fetal heart rate (FHR) monitor and a real-time ultrasound machine to assess five biophysical variables:

1. Fetal breathing movements
2. Discrete body or limb movements
3. Fetal tone
4. FHR
5. Amniotic fluid volume

The technique and interpretation are described in Suggested further reading. BPP scoring can predict adverse outcome more precisely than can NST, but its use does not seem to improve that outcome. It is, however, of value in women at high risk of fetal problems mainly because a normal result is reassuring.

5. Doppler studies

This sophisticated ultrasonic technique assesses flow velocity waveforms in blood vessels. *It does not measure flow directly*, although it is commonly assumed to do so. Umbilical artery, maternal 'utero-placental' vessels, maternal uterine artery and fetal aortic and cerebral artery flow velocity waveforms have been studied. Umbilical arterial waveform assessment may be of value in cases at increased risk of adverse outcome. The others have not yet been adequately assessed. In general therefore, Doppler ultrasound should not be part of routine clinical practice until it has been more widely tested in well-designed trials.

6. Placental architecture
A method has been described for grading the placenta antenatally by ultrasound looking at the extent and distribution of echogenic calcium deposits within it.
The clinical value of this is undetermined because it has not been adequately tested.

INTRAUTERINE GROWTH RETARDATION (IUGR)

This is erroneously taken to be synonymous with light-for-gestational-age defined as birthweight less than the tenth (or more rigorously the fifth or third) percentile for gestational age and sex. Many infants below the tenth percentile are appropriately grown and healthy. Some whose weight lies above the tenth percentile have not achieved their full growth potential and are therefore growth-retarded.
Definition — failure to achieve full growth potential. Causes:
1. Genetic — chromosomal
2. Congenital malformations
3. Multiple pregnancy
4. Chronic maternal or fetal infections
5. Maternal smoking
6. Factors affecting placental perfusion, e.g. high altitude, maternal disease processes, pre-eclampsia; in these cases head growth is relatively spared, i.e. IUGR is asymmetrical.

In causes 1–5, both head and body size are reduced, i.e. IUGR is symmetrical. The prognosis for infants with IUGR depends on the aetiology, gestational age and degree of accompanying hypoxia. For neonatal problems see pp. 159–62.

SUGGESTED FURTHER READING

Ambrose S E, Petrie R H 1989 Antenatal detection of fetal compromise. Fetal Medicine Review 1: 27–41
Enkin M, Keirse M J N C, Chalmers I 1989 Effective care in pregnancy and childbirth. Oxford University Press, Oxford
Stirrat G M 1985 Pocket consultant in obstetrics. 2nd edn. Blackwell Scientific Publications, Oxford
Turnbull A, Chamberlain G (eds) 1989 Obstetrics. Churchill Livingstone, Edinburgh
Yagel S, Adoni A, Omman S, Wax Y, Hochner-Celniker D 1986 British Journal of Obstetrics and Gynaecology 93: 109–115

Drugs and pregnancy

DRUGS USED FOR THERAPY

The following are among the factors which must be considered when prescribing any drug during pregnancy and lactation:

1. Most drugs cross the placenta and are excreted in breast milk
2. In the first trimester there is a theoretical risk of congenital malformation. Very few drugs, however, have been conclusively shown to be teratogenic
3. Fetal growth and development can be impaired by drugs taken during the second and third trimesters
4. Some drugs given close to term or during labour may affect the neonate
5. Even non-prescription drugs, such as cough medicines (containing iodides), can be harmful; ointments applied to the nipple may be harmful if ingested by the infant

Principles for prescribing during pregnancy and lactation

1. Drugs should be prescribed for a pregnant woman only when the indications are clear and specific, and the expected benefit to the mother is greater than the risk to the fetus
2. If at all possible, avoid all drugs in the first trimester (even non-prescription drugs)
3. Prescribe drugs which have been well tried in pregnancy in preference to newer preparations
4. Use the smallest effective dose for the shortest therapeutic time

Guide to prescribing during pregnancy and lactation

1. *Drugs to be avoided totally*, either because risks outweigh therapeutic benefit or because safer alternatives are available:

Drug	*Effect*
ACE inhibitors	Skull ossification defect, oligohydramnios, neonatal hypotension and anuria
Anti-androgens (cyproterone acetate)	Genital malformation in males; later sexual dysfunction?

Drug	*Effect*
Barbiturates as hypnotics and sedatives (especially in labour and when breast-feeding)	Severe neonatal respiratory depression
Diazoxide	Hyperglycaemia; alopecia in newborn
Di-ethyl stilboestrol	Associated with vaginal carcinoma and other problems in offspring
Danazol	Virilisation of female
Iodides and ^{131}iodine	Fetal hypothyroidism
Live viral vaccines (rubella, smallpox, measles, polio and yellow fever)	Viruses cross the placenta
Methotrexate	Teratogenic
Oral hypoglycaemic agents	Neonatal hypoglycaemia
Oral progestogens	Virilisation of female fetus
Phenindione	Congenital malformations: fetal and neonatal haemorrhage
Streptomycin	Oto-toxicity
Tetracyclines	Affects fetal teeth and bones
Vitamin A in high doses (isotretinoin, etretinate)	Strongly teratogenic

2. *Drugs best avoided*:

<table>
<tr><th>In first trimester</th><th>Throughout pregnancy</th><th>During lactation</th></tr>
<tr><td>Antacids</td><td colspan="2">Amiodarone</td></tr>
<tr><td>Iron supplements</td><td>Benzodiazepines</td><td>Chloramphenicol</td></tr>
<tr><td>Metronidazole</td><td>Clofibrate</td><td>Laxatives</td></tr>
<tr><td>Salicylates</td><td></td><td></td></tr>
<tr><td>Sodium valproate</td><td>Diuretics</td><td></td></tr>
<tr><td></td><td>Ergotamine</td><td></td></tr>
<tr><td></td><td>Hypnotics</td><td></td></tr>
<tr><td></td><td colspan="2">Iodide cough mixtures</td></tr>
<tr><td></td><td>Probenecid</td><td></td></tr>
<tr><td></td><td>Propranolol</td><td></td></tr>
<tr><td></td><td>Prostaglandin-synthetase inhibitors</td><td></td></tr>
</table>

3. *Drugs to be used under specialist supervision and with unequivocal indications*

Anticonvulsants	
Anti-thyroid drugs	Hypotensive agents
Anti-viral agents	Lithium carbonate
Aminoglycoside antibiotics	Systemic corticosteroids
Cytotoxic drugs	Warfarin sodium

It must not be assumed that drugs not mentioned are safe. More detailed information can be found in Suggested further reading.

DRUGS OF ABUSE

1. *Maternal cigarette smoking* is associated with an increased risk of microcephaly, facial clefts, and low birthweight. It is probably the commonest preventable risk marker for late fetal death. There is a long-term relation between smoking in pregnancy and the intellectual development of the offspring. These effects are due to (i) a direct feto-placental effect of nicotine and its metabolites, and (ii) reduced fetal oxygenation
2. *Alcohol and pregnancy*. Excessive chronic alcohol ingestion is usually defined as >80 g/day (equivalent to at least eight large glasses of wine). It is associated with a group of fetal problems — the fetal alcohol syndrome. The incidence in North America is between 1 and 2/1000 births. It is less common in the UK despite a high level of alcohol abuse in society. The principal features of the fetal alcohol syndrome are: mental retardation, growth retardation and facial anomalies. Other congenital anomalies are also said to be more common. The effects of moderate alcohol ingestion (up to 40 g/day) are much more difficult to assess because: (i) an accurate drink history is difficult to obtain, and (ii) its effects are compounded by other variables such as smoking, social class, age and parity. There may be some women in whom the fetus is particularly susceptible to damage from even moderate alcohol ingestion
3. *Marijuana* smoking is associated with a reduction in birthweight. This could be due to:
   (i) The direct effect of cannabis
   (ii) Reduced fetal oxygenation
   (iii) Increase in maternal heart rate and blood pressure
   There may also be a synergistic action with cocaine
4. *Heroin abuse* is associated with an increased risk of pre-term delivery and low birthweight. A significant number of newborns have signs of withdrawal — up to 85% if mothers injected heroin, and over 30% for those who smoked it
5. *Cocaine* abuse causes a large number of pregnancy complications such as miscarriage, abruption, growth

retardation, premature delivery, fetal distress and congenital malformations. It affects the neurobehavioural development of the infant and is associated with an increased incidence of sudden infant death. Many of these effects can be attributed to its marked vasoconstrictive effects on uteroplacental and fetal vessels

SUGGESTED FURTHER READING

Beeley L, Stirrat G M (eds) 1986 Prescribing in pregnancy. In: Clinics in obstetrics and gynaecology. Saunders, Eastbourne, Vol 13, No. 2

British National Formulary 1990 Number 20. BMA and Pharmaceutical Society of Great Britain, London

Stirrat G M 1985 Pocket consultant in obstetrics. 2nd edn. Blackwell, Oxford

Medical and surgical problems in pregnancy

HYPERTENSION AND RENAL DISEASE

Relevant physiological changes in pregnancy

Cardiovascular system

Plasma volume increases from early in pregnancy to its maximum at 32 to 34 weeks' gestation. The mean increase in primigravidae is about 1250 ml (48%), and in multigravidae it is about 1500 ml. (58%). From 34 weeks the volume falls by 200 to 300 ml. It returns to non-pregnant levels by six to eight weeks postpartum. The following table illustrates some other general haemodynamic changes.

	Before pregnancy	*Pregnancy (weeks)*				*After pregnancy (12 weeks)*
		8	16	24	36	
Cardiac output (l/min)	4	5 (25% ↑)	← 6 (50% ↑) →			4
Stroke volume (ml)	65	← 80 (20% ↑) →				Returned to normal
Heart rate (beats/min)	65	70 (8% ↑)			80 (20% ↑)	70
Systemic vascular resistance (dynes/cm/sec^{-5})	1380	970 (30% ↓)	← 930 → (33% ↓)		1210 (12% ↓)	1530 (10% ↑)

The mechanisms producing these changes are poorly understood (see below and Suggested further reading). Central venous pressure does not change in pregnancy, but peripheral venodilatation occurs from about 28 weeks' gestation.

Pulmonary haemodynamics

	Before pregnancy	Pregnancy (weeks)			
		8	16	24	36
Pulmonary blood flow (l/min)	5	6 (20% ↑)	← 7 (40% ↑) →		
Pulmonary arterial pressure (PAP) (mmHg)	16	16	18 (12% ↑)	19 (19% ↑)	18 (12% ↑)
Pulmonary vascular resistance (PAP/flow)	3.4	2.6 (24% ↓)	2.5 (26% ↓)	2.7 (20% ↓)	2.5 (26% ↓)

Pulmonary capillary wedge pressure (PCWP) does not change because of physiological ventricular dilatation.

Blood pressure (BP)

BP is proportional to cardiac output and systemic vascular resistance. Since the fall in the latter is greater than the rise in the former, the systolic blood pressure (SBP) falls slightly in early pregnancy but rises again in late pregnancy. The diastolic blood pressure (DBP) is well below non-pregnant levels from early in pregnancy. It returns to those levels after 30 to 32 weeks' gestation.

An important factor in changing vascular resistance and controlling BP is the balance between vasodilatory prostacyclin (PGI_2) and vasoconstrictive thromboxane A_2 (TXA_2), but other mechanisms are also involved (see Suggested further reading).

The normally pregnant woman is relatively refractory to vasopressor agents, i.e. her BP does not rise in response to a small dose of a vasopressor (cf. pre-eclampsia p. 61).

Urinary system

1. Anatomical changes. The renal tracts begin to dilate by 10 weeks of pregnancy (right > left). These changes are due partly to mechanical pressure — but not solely to it. The role of progesterone is now questioned. Dilatation persists for 12–16 weeks after delivery
2. Renal haemodynamics and function. The major changes are roughly as shown in the following table.

Total body water increases by 6–8 litres with retention of sodium. The passage of normal urine volumes in the face of low

	Non-pregnant	Early pregnancy	Late pregnancy
Renal blood flow (ml/min)	480	840(75% ↑)	770(60% ↑)
Glomerular filtration rate (GFR)			
Inulin clearance (ml/min)	105	163(55% ↑)	169(60% ↑)
Creatinine clearance (24 h; ml/min)	94	136(45% ↑)	144(20% ↑)
Plasma			
Creatinine μmol/l	77	60(22% ↓)	64(17% ↓)
Urea mmol/l	4.3	3.0(30% ↓)	2.8(35% ↓)
Urate μmol/l	245	190(22% ↓)	270(10 ↑)
Osmolality mosm/kg	290	280(4% ↓)	280(4% ↓)

plasma osmolality and a raised extracellular fluid volume is unique to pregnancy. It is due to a resetting of the osmoreceptors and the maintenance of arginine vasopressin (AVP) secretion.

Hypertensive disorders in pregnancy

Definitions

Hypertension — two consecutive measurements of diastolic blood pressure (DBP) ⩾90 mmHg 4 or more hours apart *or* one measurement ⩾110 mmHg. The DBP is taken at the 'point of muffling' (Korotkoff phase IV) in women lying on their side with a 15° to 30° tilt. The use of systolic blood pressure (SBP) or the calculation of mean arterial pressure does not add to the prognostic significance and is more complicated. A DBP of 90 mmHg corresponds to the point at which the perinatal mortality rate begins to rise in population studies, and is approximately the mean + 3 SD in mid-pregnancy, the mean + 2 SD from 34 to 37 weeks, and the mean + 1 SD at term. The significance of the same level of hypertension, therefore, varies with the stage in pregnancy at which it is recorded.

Severe hypertension — a DBP ⩾120 mmHg on one occasion *or* a DBP ⩾110 mmHg on two consecutive occasions 4 or more hours apart.

Proteinuria

1. A 24-hour urine collection containing ⩾300 mg protein
2. Two random MSU or catheter specimens with a protein/creatinine index

$$\frac{(10 \times \text{protein mg/l})}{(\text{creatinine nmol/l})} \geqslant 300 \text{ mg}$$

(i) 2 + (1 g albumin/l) or more on reagent strip or sulphosalicyclic acid 'cold test'.

(ii) 1 + (0.3 g albumin/l) or more if urinary SG < 1030 because the dilution of urine affects the protein concentration

Classification for medical audit

Gestational hypertension and/or proteinuria
Hypertension and/or proteinuria developing during pregnancy, labour or the puerperium in a previously normotensive non-proteinuric woman subdivided into:
Gestational hypertension (without proteinuria)
Gestational proteinuria (without hypertension)
Gestational proteinuric hypertension (pre-eclampsia)
Each of these can develop during pregnancy, in labour, or in the puerperium.

Chronic hypertension and chronic renal disease
Hypertension and/or proteinuria in a woman with either chronic hypertension or chronic renal disease present before, diagnosed during, or persisting after pregnancy subdivided into:
Chronic hypertension (without proteinuria)
Chronic renal disease — proteinuria with/without hypertension
Chronic hypertension with superimposed pre-eclampsia (proteinuria developing for the first time in pregnancy in a woman with known chronic hypertension)

Women with hypertension and/or proteinuria when first seen before 20 weeks' gestation (who do not have a hydatidiform mole) are classified under this heading.

Unclassified hypertension and/or proteinuria
Hypertension and/or proteinuria found either:

1. At first booking examination at or after 20 weeks of pregnancy in a woman without known chronic hypertension or chronic renal disease, *or*
2. During labour, pregnancy or the puerperium but where insufficient information is available to permit classification subdivided into:
   Unclassified hypertension (without proteinuria)
   Unclassified proteinuria (without hypertension)
   Unclassified proteinuric hypertension (pre-eclampsia)

The classification in pregnancy is provisional and should be reviewed at the end of the puerperium.

Pre-eclampsia
Pre-eclampsia is a multi-system disorder peculiar to pregnancy, of unknown aetiology, usually characterised by hypertension,

renal impairment, and fluid retention, and often accompanied by proteinuria and some degree of intravascular coagulation.

Primary pathology
Abnormal maternal adaptation to the presence of trophoblast. This is not specific to pre-eclampsia and can also occur in 'idiopathic' IUGR. The primary consequences are:

1. Relative lack of trophoblast infiltration of the walls of maternal spiral arterioles during development of the placenta
2. Failure of normal development of the uteroplacental circulation
3. Aggregation of platelets, fibrin and lipid-laden macrophages ('acute atherosis') within unadapted spiral arterioles

The mother's physiological adaptation to pregnancy is also abnormal. For example:

1. Plasma volume does not expand normally. The net effect is a reduced maternal plasma volume
2. Prostanoid production is abnormal. One example is a relative reduction of endothelial production of prostacyclin (PGI_2) compared to thromboxane. This affects systemic vascular resistance as evidenced by:
   (i) Continued responsiveness to vasopressors (cf. normal pregnancy p. 58)
   (ii) The development of hypertension

There is a resulting cascade effect on virtually every system in the body. Among these effects are

1. *Vascular endothelium* — generalised changes seem to occur, and specific effects are seen in a variety of organs (discussed below). The imbalance between PGI_2 and thromboxane is an example of failure of maternal adaptation which predisposes to pathology. Antibodies to vascular endothelium have been detected in severe cases and may mediate some of the damage
2. *The kidney* — the glomerular endothelial cells swell, blocking the capillaries. This 'glomerular endotheliosis' is characteristic but not pathognomonic. Pre-eclampsia is the commonest cause of heavy proteinuria in pregnancy and can cause nephrotic syndrome (p. 72). A rise in plasma urate is an early feature of pre-eclampsia
3. *Coagulation* — the physiological changes in the clotting system in pregnancy are outlined on p. 93. Intravascular coagulation to a slight degree is common but can be severe in pre-eclampsia as manifested by
   (i) platelet turnover is increased which can result in larger platelets on a blood film and a fall in platelet count which can be severe in some cases (see below)
   (ii) DIC is a rare but serious end point in some cases

(iii) Haemolysis can occur due to fibrinogen-associated red cell aggregation

4. *The liver* — hepato-cellular damage can occur due to fibrin deposits in the sinusoids. It can be detected by elevation of liver enzymes in maternal serum. The epigastric pain and vomiting associated with fulminating pre-eclampsia are due to effects on the liver. In some cases, jaundice and severe liver damage can follow, often out of proportion to other signs and symptoms. DIC is also present. The HELLP syndrome (haemolysis, elevated liver enzymes, and low platelets) is a dangerous presentation of pre-eclampsia and must be considered in severe cases. Hepatic encephalopathy can occur and it has a high maternal mortality. *Liver involvement must be considered in all cases of severe pre-eclampsia.* Early recognition has a good maternal and fetal prognosis; late recognition has a poor prognosis
5. *Cardio-pulmonary effects.* Severe pre-eclampsia is a high cardiac output state with inappropriately high systemic vascular resistance. Left ventricular function is hyperdynamic. Cardiac failure can therefore complicate the most severe cases. Pulmonary oedema may arise due to an imbalance between a reduced colloid osmotic pressure and the pulmonary capillary wedge pressure. *It can also be precipitated by intravenous fluid overload during treatment without proper monitoring* (see p. 68)
6. *Central nervous system* — among the signs of CNS involvement are atypical headache, hyper-reflexia, visual disturbances, and ankle clonus. Vasoconstriction of cerebral vessels occurs, probably as a protective mechanism against severe hypertension. At a mean arterial pressure of about 130 to 150 mmHg this mechanism begins to fail, and small vessel walls are damaged and disrupted. This leads to cerebral oedema, haemorrhages and infarcts — all associated with *eclampsia* (see p. 68) a major cause of maternal death
7. *Feto/placental effects.* Pre-eclampsia is the commonest cause of:
   (i) IUGR in non-malformed infants
   (ii) Elective pre-term delivery

   Perinatal death is increased:
   (i) In severe disease of early onset (10- to 15-fold)
   (ii) When eclampsia occurs

Maternal mortality and pre-eclampsia/eclampsia
Hypertensive diseases of pregnancy and pulmonary embolus shared first place as causes of maternal death in England and Wales (1982–84). Of the 25 women who died, the causes of death were as shown in the following table.

	Pre-eclampsia	*Eclampsia*	*Total*
Cerebral haemorrhage	7	6	13(52%)
Cerebral infarction/'softening'	2	2	4(16%)
Cerebral oedema	1	3	4(16%)
Pulmonary oedema (i.v. fluid overload)	1	2	3(12%)
Hepatic necrosis	1	–	1(4%)

Predisposing factors

1. *Primigravidity*. The incidence of proteinuric pre-eclampsia in a first pregnancy is around 6%. It occurs in about 2% of all second pregnancies, rising to 12% if proteinuric pre-eclampsia (with IUGR) was present in the first, and falling to 0.7% if the first was a singleton, normotensive pregnancy. Pregnancy by a new partner may increase the risk to that of a first pregnancy. No protection is offered by an early spontaneous or induced abortion.
2. *Genetic*. Pre-eclampsia is more likely among women whose mother or sisters developed it also. Inheritance can be explained by maternal homozygosity for a recessive gene which may be linked to HLA-DR4.

   It is also more common when there is a strong family history of hypertension, other cardiovascular disorders or auto-immune disease. There is no significant racial preponderance
3. *Medical*. Pre-existing hypertension and diabetes mellitus predispose
4. *Socio-economic*. The increasing incidence as socio-economic status deteriorates is associated with poor maternal nutrition and short stature. The incidence is lower in women who smoke, but the fetal outlook is poor in smokers who develop pre-eclampsia
5. *Obstetric*. Multiple pregnancy and hydatidiform mole can be associated with very early and severe pre-eclampsia. It also tends to occur when hydrops fetalis (rhesus and non-rhesus) is present

Management of pre-eclampsia

The principles are:

1. Prompt diagnosis
2. Awareness of serious nature of the condition in its severe form without over reacting to mild disease
3. Agreed guidelines for admission to hospital, investigation, and antihypertensive therapy

4. Well-timed delivery to pre-empt serious maternal or fetal complications
5. Postnatal follow up and counselling for future pregnancies

Clinical observation and investigation
Examination (over and above routine):
1. Palpation of the femoral pulses (to exclude coarctation of aorta)
2. Exclude kidney enlargement
3. Look for hyper-reflexia and ankle clonus
4. Check optic fundi for silver wiring, arterio-venous nipping, exudates and haemorrhage

Laboratory investigation
1. *Urine microscopy and culture.* Bacterial counts of $10^5/mm^3$ are significant (repeat if 10^4–$10^5/mm^3$)
2. *Proteinuria* — see p. 59.
3. *Serum urate* levels increase early in pre-eclampsia. Levels > 350 μmol/l are abnormal in pregnancy but gradually increasing levels are more significant
4. *Serum urea and creatinine.* Rising levels are significant but not so sensitive indicators of pre-eclampsia as uric acid. The upper limits of normal in pregnancy are 5 mmol/l for serum urea and 100 μmol/l for creatinine, but trends are even more important than specific levels
5. *Creatinine clearance*
6. *Urinary catecholamines or vanillyl mandelic acid (VMA-a catecholamine metabolite)* are raised in the presence of a phaeochromocytoma (see p. 84)
7. *Platelet count* gradually falls if disseminated intravascular coagulation is occurring.
8. *Liver function* — this should be checked once persistent proteinuria is present, or if platelet count is significantly reduced. Coagulation studies should be carried out if platelet count is reduced and in severe disease.
9. Tests of fetal growth and well-being (see p. 45)

Management of mild hypertension
The principles are:
1. Bedrest is usually effective in reducing mild hypertension
2. The use of sedatives or tranquillisers is contra-indicated
3. Antihypertensive therapy is not indicated (see below)
4. Uncomplicated hypertension is suitable for careful supervision at home by the primary health care team
5 Admission to hospital is indicated when:
   (i) SBP is 160 and/or DBP 100 mmHg or greater. The tendency to ignore blood pressures of the above order because readings taken 5 to 10 minutes later are

significantly lower is to be deprecated. The tendency to develop hypertension has been demonstrated and that suggests the possibility of increased risk
(ii) Proteinuria is detected in a clean (i.e. mid-stream) urine sample in the absence of a urinary infection
(iii) The patient is symptomatic with e.g. visual disturbances, unusual headache, epigastric pain, vomiting or twitching
(iv) There is clinical evidence of intrauterine growth retardation
(v) Tests of fetal welfare have deteriorated (see p. 45)
(vi) A previous bad obstetric history suggests that closer surveillance would be worthwhile

Management of severe hypertension
The maternal risks of cerebrovascular accident and of left ventricular or renal failure begin to increase significantly when hypertension is severe. The choice has then to be made between delivery and antihypertensive therapy. Among the factors to be considered are:
1. *Gestational age* — it is seldom justified to commence long-term oral therapy from 34 weeks
2. Availability of *intensive neonatal care facilities*
3. Symptoms and signs suggesting *impending eclampsia*

Treatment neither influences the progression of underlying pre-eclampsia nor significantly improves fetal outcome. It helps to protect the mother and enables many pregnancies to continue that otherwise would be ended because of maternal risk.

Control of acute severe hypertension
There is no consensus on the optimum acute treatment. The important objective is to reduce the blood pressure to safe levels (but not too low!). The table below (p. 66) gives a guide to the best options. For more detailed discussion see Suggested further reading.

Longer-term control of severe hypertension
The indications for the need for longer-term control are:
1. DBP $\geq$ 100 mgHg
2. Pregnancy $\leq$ 34 weeks
3. Fetal and maternal state otherwise good

Treatment options are shown in the table on page 67.

Among the drugs best avoided in pregnancy are:
Diazoxide — can produce profound maternal hypotension, and fetal alopecia
Atenolol — may have deleterious fetal effect
Angiotensin converting enzymes (ACE) inhibitors — have deleterious fetal effects

Table A Control of acute severe hypertension

Drug	*Action*	*Regimen*	*Benefits*	*Disadvantages*	*Comments*
Hydralazine	Non-specific vasodilator	5 mg by slow i.v. injection, then at 5 mg/h doubling every 30 min to max of 40 mg/h until BP controlled	Effective	Causes tachycardia and severe headache; may mimic impending eclampsia	Not ideal for long-term control of severe hypertension
Labetalol	Beta > alpha adrenergic blocking agent	20 mg/h doubled every 30 min to max 160 mg/h until control obtained	Lowers BP smoothly	Some women do not respond (genetic effect?)	
Nifedipine	Calcium channel blocking agent; vasolidator	5–10 mg b.d. up to 40 mg	Good control of BP	Can cause severe headaches	Not recommended in combination with beta blockers or magnesium sulphate and see table B

Table B Longer-term control of severe hypertension

Drug	*Action*	*Regimen*	*Benefits*	*Disadvantages*	*Comments*
Alpha-methyl dopa	Central effect	500 mg orally then 250 mg 6-hourly (to max 750 mg)	Well tested and safe; can be combined with oral hydralazine	Causes initial drowsiness, and postural hypotension; crosses placenta but effect not significant	Less used because of fashion
Oxprenolol	Beta-blocking agent	80 to 480 mg daily, orally	Good control of BP	May cause bronchospasm if patient asthmatic; crosses placenta	Beneficial effect on fetal weight not confirmed
Labetalol	Beta > alpha blocking agent	100 to 200 mg 8-hourly, orally	Good control of BP	Some women do not respond; can cause postural hypotension	
Hydralazine	Vasodilator	25 to 75 mg 6-hourly, orally	Best used with methyl dopa which blocks some of its side effects	See above	Not first-line therapy
Nifedipine	Calcium channel blocking agent and vasodilator	5 to 10 mg b.d.; up to 40 mg can be given by slow-release tablets	Good control orally	Can cause headache, flushing, ankle swelling with longer-term use	Use promising but not yet fully assessed

Diuretics — contra-indicated for pre-eclampsia because they further reduce circulating blood volume

Timing of delivery
The most common grounds for delivery are:

1. Progressive fetal compromise (i.e. when the baby is safer delivered)
2. Unacceptable risk to maternal health, e.g. uncontrollable B.P., impending renal failure or heart failure, increasing jaundice or DIC, eclampsia (see below)

The mode of delivery (Caesarean section versus vaginal) depends on the seriousness of the situation, the gestational age and the degree of fetal/maternal compromise

Epidural analgesia is the method of choice for labour as long as a coagulation defect has been excluded. There is no need to test this in all pre-eclamptic women. The indications are persistent proteinuria accompanied by a significant reduction in platelets. Appropriate facilities for the care of the newborn infant must be available

Fluid balance and plasma volume expansion

1. Salt restriction is unnecessary
2. Diuretics are contraindicated because they aggravate hypovolaemia and can precipitate renal failure
3. Plasma volume expansion accompanied by vasodilator drugs (e.g. hydralazine) may have a role in some severe cases with the following provisos:
   (i) It must be used only in high-dependency units where invasive monitoring (e.g. to measure pulmonary capillary wedge pressure — PCWP) is available
   (ii) Only small volumes (e.g. haemaccel 200–600 ml) are necessary
   (iii) *Blind therapy is very dangerous and can lead to pulmonary oedema and death*
   (iv) CVP monitoring is not adequate. Measurement of PCWP is necessary (CVP does not correlate with PCWP when the former is >6 mmHg)
4. Restriction of i.v. fluids to less than 1 litre following delivery of women with severe pre-eclampsia reduces the risk of pulmonary oedema without affecting renal function

Imminent eclampsia and eclampsia
Eclampsia is defined as fits occurring during or shortly after pregnancy no matter the level of blood pressure or other finding unless the patient is already known to have epilepsy or other pre-existing disease associated with fits. In half of the cases fits occur before labour. Postpartum fits usually occur within 24 hours of delivery, but rarely occur up to 3 weeks later.

Eclampsia is still a major contributor to maternal mortality (see p. 155). In addition to hypertension the symptoms and signs suggesting impending eclampsia are:

1. Unusual headache — persistent, severe, generalised (but may be occipital or frontal)
2. Visual disturbance — e.g. blurring, flashes or spots, photophobia
3. Restlessness, agitation
4. Epigastric pain, nausea and vomiting
5. Sudden severe hypertension and proteinuria (but these may not occur)
6. Hyper-reflexia and clonus
7. Retinal oedema, haemorrhages and even papilloedema
8. Oliguria

Management

1. *Prevention or control of convulsions.* Different drugs should be considered to prevent and to treat convulsions. Intravenous diazepam, 0.8% chlormethiazole, or phenytoin sodium can be used (intramuscular diazepam and phenytoin are ineffective). If diazepam is used consciousness is not lost completely but the fetus may be depressed after birth. Chlormethiazole does not depress cough reflexes or respiratory centres. Phenytoin has no CNS sedative action.

   Intravenous and intramuscular magnesium sulphate has retained its popularity in the USA for the management of eclampsia. It reduces neuromuscular irritability and causes cerebral depression. The margin of safety is not large. Diazepam is probably the treatment of choice to treat fits. Magnesium sulphate and phenytoin can be used to prevent them.

   Status eclampticus — if the convulsions cannot be controlled by the above it may be necessary to paralyse the patient with a muscle relaxant and use artificial ventilation.
2. *Control of hypertension* (see p. 65)
3. *General management.* Patency of the airway must be maintained and oxygen given as necessary
   A urinary catheter should be inserted to monitor urine output
   Check for disorders of electrolyte balance and disseminated intravascular coagulation
4. *Delivery of the infant.* Caesarean section is the method of choice but only when the eclampsia is under control. If eclampsia supervenes when the patient is well advanced in labour vaginal delivery may be possible.

Prevention of pre-eclampsia?

Pre-eclampsia and/or IUGR may be preventable in women at high risk of developing them by daily low-dose aspirin. This suppresses production of thromboxane A_2 by platelets without significantly affecting prostacyclin. The relative imbalance found in pre-eclampsia is, therefore, corrected. Several small trials have suggested benefit but the results of a large multicentre trial are awaited. Routine low-dose aspirin therapy cannot be justified. The longer-term effects on mother and fetus are still not known.

Long-term outlook
Severely pre-eclamptic/eclamptic primigravidae are *not* at increased risk of developing chronic hypertension (given that there is not pre-existing hypertension). Later chronic H/T is, on the other hand, relatively common among severely pre-eclamptic multiparous women because it is their latent hypertension which predisposes them to pre-eclampsia in the first place.

Chronic (pre-existing) hypertension
Possible causes include:

1. Essential hypertension — the outlook is good in this condition but pre-eclampsia may supervene. Management of the hypertension is as described above.
2. Coarctation of the aorta
3. Renal hypertension — this is discussed below
4. Phaeochromocytoma — see p. 84
5. Autoimmune connective tissue disorders — see p. 86
6. Some drugs, e.g. corticosteroids, MAO inhibitors, phenacetin (secondary to effect on kidney)

SUGGESTED FURTHER READING

Davey D A 1985 Hypertensive disorders of pregnancy. In: Studd J (ed) Progress in obstetrics and gynaecology. Churchill Livingstone, Edinburgh, p. 89

MacGillivray I 1983 Pre-eclampsia. Saunders, London

Redman C W G 1989 Hypertension in pregnancy. In: Turnbull A C, Chamberlain G (eds) Obstetrics. Churchill Livingstone, Edinburgh, pp. 515–541

Rubin P C 1986 Treatment of hypertension in pregnancy. In: Beeley L, Stirrat G M (eds) Clinics in obstetrics and gynaecology, Vol 13, No. 2

Stirrat G M 1985 Pocket consultant in obstetrics. 2nd edn. Blackwell, Oxford (contains detailed regimes)

URINARY TRACT INFECTIONS

Asymptomatic bacteriuria

Bacteriuria is significant when the cultured urine contains $>$100 000 organisms/ml. Asymptomatic bacteriuria occurs in about 5% of pregnancies; *Escherichia coli* (*E. coli*) is the infecting organism in 90% of cases. Pregnancy does not predispose to it but it progresses to acute pyelonephritis in a greater proportion (25–40%) of pregnant women. Routine culture of a mid-stream urine (MSU) should be performed at booking because:

1. Detection and treatment prevents at least two-thirds of the cases of acute pyelonephritis
2. Maternal anaemia and IUGR may be more common in untreated cases

Recurrent bacteriuria is common.

Acute pyelonephritis

This usually presents as a febrile illness with loin pain and vomiting. It needs to be differentiated from other causes of an acute abdomen. It is associated with pre-term labour and, sometimes, fetal death. Blood cultures should be taken in severe cases. *E. coli* is the commonest infecting organism. Treatment with appropriate antibiotic should begin while urine culture and sensitivity results are awaited. It should continue in full therapeutic doses for 3 to 6 weeks. Thereafter urine culture should be performed from each antenatal visit. If it recurs consider maintenance antibacterial therapy for the remainder of pregnancy and for 2 weeks postpartum.

Chronic renal disease

Pregnancy *per se* does not usually adversely affect most renal diseases with the possible exception of membrano-proliferative glomerulonephritis and lupus nephropathy.

The increased risk of urinary infection in pregnancy can lead to exacerbation of chronic pyelonephritis.

The outcome of pregnancy is proportional to the severity of renal impairment rather than specific diseases.

Pre-pregnancy counselling

Pregnancy is not advisable in women whose plasma creatinine levels are ≥200 μmol/l and whose DBP is ≥90 mmHg. Most women with severe renal impairment are amenorrhoeic and infertile. Among the renal diseases seen in pregnancy are:

1. Chronic pyelonephritis — good prognosis if renal function adequate and normotensive
2. Chronic glomerulonephritis — patients more liable to develop superadded pre-eclampsia
3. Polycystic kidneys — prognosis depends on renal function and level of BP
4. Auto-immune connective tissue disease nephropathy — see p. 86
5. Diabetic nephropathy (see p. 78)

Regular antenatal assessment should be carried out of:
1. Maternal blood pressure, renal function and urine cultures
2. Fetal growth and well-being (see p. 45)

Nephrotic syndrome
— heavy proteinuria (>3.5 g/24 h), with hypoalbuminaemia and gross generalised oedema. The commonest cause in late pregnancy is pre-eclampsia. If it occurs before 32 weeks' gestation a high-protein diet can be given and salt-free albumen infusions considered after seeking advice from a nephrologist. Steroids should not be given unless a biopsy-proven diagnosis suggests that they would be beneficial (e.g. membranoproliferative glomerulonephritis). Diuretics are contraindicated.

Renal and ureteric calculi
If this diagnosis is suspected, intravenous urography is indicated if two of the following are present:
1. Microscopic haematuria
2. Recurrent symptoms referable to urinary tract
3. Sterile urine culture when symptoms suggest pyelonephritis.

Management is initially conservative, with hydration, antibiotics and analgesia. Surgery is rarely necessary.

Renal allografts and pregnancy
Chronic haemodialysis is associated with infertility, and successful pregnancy is uncommon in women receiving this treatment.
Renal transplantation restores fertility in proportion to reproductive age and allograft function.

Pre-pregnancy counselling
The following criteria are guides to the timing of pregnancy:
1. At least 18 months since transplant
2. Renal function stable, with no proteinuria and plasma creatinine ≤200 μmol/l
3. Normotensive (or nearly so)
4. No evidence of graft rejection
5. Immunosuppressive therapy at maintenance levels

Ante-natal care should be hospital-based in a joint clinic involving obstetrician and nephrologist. In addition to routine, maternal assessment should include screening for anaemia, any infection, and superadded pre-eclampsia. Graft rejection is no more or less common. Renal ultrasonography may be helpful in its detection. Immunosuppressive therapy should be maintained. The effects of cyclosporin therapy in pregnancy need to be evaluated. Vaginal delivery should be aimed for. Caesarean section is indicated for obstetric reasons only. Fetal outcome is surprisingly good, although pre-term delivery (elective and spontaneous) and IUGR are more common. Congenital malformations are not more common. Neonates may be more prone to viral or other infections. There is disagreement as to whether breast feeding is or is not to be encouraged.

Post-partum contraception poses a problem. On balance, a low-dose combined pill (see p. 202) may be best as long as surveillance is frequent.

SUGGESTED FURTHER READING

Brudenell M, Wilde P L 1984 Medical and surgical problems in obstetrics. Wright, Bristol

Turnbull A C, Chamberlain G 1989 Obstetrics. Churchill Livingstone, Edinburgh

ANAEMIA

The haemoglobin (Hb) concentration falls during pregnancy (but not normally below 10.4 g/dl) because the physiological increase in plasma volume outstrips that of the red cell mass.

The average requirement for iron is about 4 mg/day increasing as the pregnancy progresses. Although the normal diet contains up to 25 mg/day of iron only about 10% of this is absorbed. Iron stores fall, therefore, during pregnancy. The first effect is a fall in serum ferritin to around 6 μg/l by 28 weeks. Hb does not fall, and microcytic erythrocytes do not appear for several weeks after the stores are exhausted.

The routine policy for supplementation of all pregnant women with iron and folate is now disputed.

Routine supplementation with iron and folate

Points for	*Points against*
Iron stores become exhausted in most pregnant women	This physiological change is usually of no clinical relevance
Anaemia is associated with a variety of adverse outcomes	Most cases can be detected and treated
Routine therapy is cheaper than identifying women at most risk	Compliance with routine prescription is not good
Routine therapy raises Hb levels	Iron therapy has side-effects in some patients

The writer favours routine supplementation with 100 mg iron and 300 μg folate daily.

Iron deficiency
The blood film is hypochromic and microcytic. MCH is decreased; serum ferritin levels are low (< 15 μg/l) and iron-binding capacity is increased.
Treatment: increase dietary sources of iron (e.g. meat, fish, eggs and spinach) and supplement with oral iron. If gastrointestinal intolerance to iron occurs change to a chelated or delayed release preparation. Parenteral iron is rarely necessary because:

1. The response is no better than to oral iron
2. The maximum response takes six weeks
3. Side-effects occur more frequently in pregnancy

An underlying folate deficiency may be unmasked by treatment.

Folate deficiency
Blood film is normochromic and macrocytic. Red cells may be nucleated and contain Howell-Jolly nuclear inclusion bodies. Check serum folate and B12 (red cell folate is low in both folate and B12 deficiency and is therefore not so helpful).
Treatment: increase dietary sources of folate (as for iron). Give 5 to 15 mg folic acid orally daily.

Vitamin B12 deficiency
Vitamin B12 deficiency is rare in pregnancy, with a higher incidence in strict vegetarians. Blood film megaloblastic. Treatment is with intramuscular vitamin B12. A daily folate supplement of 300 μg will not mask vitamin B12 deficiency.

Sickle-cell disease
For genetics see p. 34. The major problem is Hb S/S, with Hb S/C and Hb S/Thal being less common. Perinatal loss and IUGR are common.
Antenatal screening. Routine Hb electrophoresis is indicated when the indigenous or immigrant population makes the risk of haemoglobinopathy high. If routine screening is not necessary a sickling test (e.g. Sickledex) should be carried out on all individuals of African origins.
Sickling crises. Hb A and its abnormal variants function similarly when well-oxygenated but the latter polymerise when deoxygenated. The red cells become sickle-shaped and occlude vessels causing widespread vascular damage, severe pain and haemolytic anaemia.
Prevention. Folate supplements and oral bicarbonate (to increase the pH of the urine); blood transfusion (3–4 units) at 6-week intervals; prompt treatment of infection.
Treatment: exchange transfusion (2.5 l out: 3.0 l in).

Sickle-cell trait (Hb A/S)
This is usually benign, but sickling cases occur under extreme hypoxia. The Hb level tends to be lower than average. It may predispose to pyelonephritis.

The management of severe anaemia in pregnancy
If Hb is < 6.0 g/dl then consider exchange transfusion or plasmaphoresis. If Hb is between 6.0 and 8.0 g/dl then transfuse slowly with three to five units of packed cells. Use intravenous frusemide 20 mg to prevent circulatory overload.

CARDIAC DISEASE

The haemodynamic changes which occur during pregnancy (see p. 57) impose an increased burden on the mother's heart. This causes no problems for healthy women but may do so in women with cardiac disease.

Rheumatic heart disease (RHD)
The incidence of RHD has decreased dramatically over the past 25 years in most developed countries. Mitral stenosis is still the commonest and most important problem. Pregnancy has no permanent deleterious effect on RHD

Congenital heart defects (CHD)
An increasing number of women with CHD are reaching childbearing age as a result of improved medical and surgical management. Most women with acyanotic CHD tolerate pregnancy well (except severe aortic stenosis and coarctation of the aorta). Patients with uncorrected CHD, pulmonary hypertension (either primary or as part of Eisenmenger's syndrome) do badly and maternal death can occur suddenly.

Other cardiac lesions

1. Tachyarrhythmias — see below
2. Myocardial infarction — this is a rare complication of pregnancy; risk factors include smoking, hypertension, diabetes mellitus and familial hypercholesterolaemia

Pre-conception counselling
This is important for women with known heart disease because:

1. Treatment can be made optimal
2. A specific plan can be prepared for pregnancy
3. Surgery can be advised in those women in whom pregnancy would add a severe but correctable burden, e.g. tight mitral stenosis
4. Advice can be given to those women at high risk during pregnancy, e.g. Marfan's syndrome, inoperable cyanotic

heart disease, primary pulmonary hypertension, Eisenmenger's syndrome; *pregnancy may be best avoided in these conditions*

Antenatal management

Termination of pregnancy is not medically indicated, except when pulmonary hypertension in severe.

1. Arrange regular antenatal visits to obstetrician and cardiologist
2. Ensure adequate rest
3. Ban smoking
4. Prevent anaemia
5. Treat respiratory infection promptly
6. Cover dental work with antibiotics
7. Be watchful for incipient pulmonary congestion and arrhythmias

Management of labour

Induction of labour is necessary only for obstetric reasons. Vaginal prostaglandins are the method of choice because early amniotomy may increase the risk of infection. When patient starts labour with good cardiac reserve the risk of heart failure is low.

1. Aim for vaginal delivery at term
2. Cover labour with antibiotics
3. Control any infusion of parenteral fluids very strictly
4. Provide adequate analgesia — epidural anaesthesia is safe in *experienced* hands as long hypotension is avoided; it is, however contraindicated in HOCM (see below) and Eisenmenger's syndrome
5. Avoid aortocaval compression
6. Shorten the second stage by use of 'lift-out' forceps or vacuum extractor (without raising legs into lithotomy position if possible)
7. Ergometrine is best avoided
8. Do not attempt Caesarean section in the presence of heart failure
9. Have oxygen and relevant drugs *immediately* available
10. Avoid beta-sympathomimetic drugs in women with pre-existing heart disease

SPECIFIC PROBLEMS

Cardiac failure

The principles of diagnosis and treatment are the same as in the non-pregnant patient. It can occur even in young asymptomatic women with cardiac disease at any stage of pregnancy. Sudden cardiac decompensation is more likely to occur shortly after delivery.

Acute pulmonary oedema is a medical emergency which demands immediate attention.

Management

1. Nurse in semi-recumbent position, give oxygen and keep airways clear
2. Give intravenous morphine, aminophylline, frusemide and digoxin (if not previously digitalised). In labour the fetus must take second place until the situation is under control

Tachyarrythmias

Atrial fibrillation is a medical emergency requiring bed rest in hospital and digitalisation. The advice of a cardiologist must always be sought. Anticoagulation may also be indicated.

Atrial tachycardia can precipitate heart failure rapidly. It often responds to carotid sinus pressure.

Cardiac surgery and pregnancy

Anticoagulant therapy must be maintained and carefully controlled in women who have had previous cardiac surgery. Warfarin is the drug of choice here even in the first trimester. Intravenous heparin should be substituted 2 to 3 weeks before anticipated time of delivery (see p. 95).

Mitral valvotomy may be indicated during pregnancy in pure severe mitral stenosis if pulmonary congestion develops, or if there is no prompt response to medical therapy.

Hypertrophic obstructive cardiomyopathy (HOCM)

Most women with HOCM tolerate pregnancy and vaginal delivery well. This depends, however, on the severity of the left ventricular outflow tract obstruction. It is important to avoid:

1. Digoxin therapy
2. Beta-sympathomimetic drugs — some of the deaths associated with their use have been in women with undiagnosed cardiomyopathy
3. Aortocaval compression — e.g. the left lateral position should be used for delivery

Caesarean section snould be reserved for obstetric indications.

DIABETES MELLITUS (DM)

Definition

Fasting venous plasma glucose concentration ≥ 8.0 mmol/l *and* ≥11.0 mmol/l 2 hours after a 75 g oral glucose load; *or* one of these plus symptoms and signs (polydipsia, polyuria, weight loss).

Impaired glucose tolerance (IGT) is present if the fasting level is <8.0 mmol/l but rises to 8.0–10.9 mmol/l 2 hours after 75 g oral glucose load.

Antenatal screening

IGT/DM must be suspected in all women with:

1. Significant glycosuria on two occasions antenatally *or* in a single fasting urine sample
2. Mother, father or siblings with diabetes
3. Previous babies > 90th centile for gestational age and sex
4. Diabetes in a previous pregnancy
5. Previous unexpected perinatal death
6. Polyhydramnios
7. Maternal obesity (> 20% above ideal weight)

Routine antenatal screening has been recommended by some because:

1. About 30% of gestational diabetes have none of the above risk features
2. Not all women with IGT or even diabetes have persistent glycosuria
3. Glycosuria can be found in the urine of up to 50% of all pregnant women at some time

Selective or comprehensive screening can be undertaken by:

1. Random blood glucose estimations at booking and at 28 to 32 weeks. Further investigation is required for levels ≥6.4 mmol/l within 2 hours of the last meal or ≥5.8 mmol/l more than 2 hours after it
2. Estimation of blood glucose concentrations fasting and 2 hours after a 50 g glucose load. An oral 75 g GTT is indicated if fasting and/or the 2-hour levels exceed 5 and 7 mmol/l respectively

Risks associated with diabetes

1. Maternal — retinopathy, nephropathy and neuropathy may be worsened
2. Congenital malformations — there is a slight general increase in malformations related to hyperglycaemia during organogenesis — especially craniospinal and cardiac defect; sacral agenesis is a rare anomaly specifically associated with diabetes
3. Obstetric complications — e.g. polyhydramnios, pre-term labour, pre-eclampsia
4. Infections — urinary, monilial and other infections
5. Sudden unexpected fetal death (SUFD) — increased risk during the last 4 to 6 weeks of pregnancy
6. Difficult delivery — because of excess fetal growth (macrosomia)

7. Neonatal problems — birth trauma, hyaline membrane disease, hypoglycaemia, hypomagnesaemia, hypocalcaemia, jaundice

All risks are increased by poor control of diabetes (especially if keto-acidosis develops) and by inadequate obstetric supervision. Macrosomia has been reported in up to 30% of seemingly well controlled diabetics.

Management

1. *Pre-pregnancy counselling* allows:
   (i) General advice, particularly about tight diabetic control
   (ii) Planning for pregnancy (including early booking for antenatal care)
   (iii) Review of diet
   (iv) Examination of optic fundi
   (v) Establishment of good blood glucose control
2. *Antenatal care* for pre-existing diabetics should be jointly between obstetrician and physician. For optimal *diabetic* control:
   (i) Organise high-fibre diet with correct calorific intake and CHO content
   (ii) Carry out blood glucose profiles two or three times/week at home using filter-paper strips or a reflectance meter. Tests are carried out before and 2 hours after each meal and last thing at night. Pre- and post-prandial levels of <5.0 and <7.0 mmol/l respectively are ideal
   (iii) Regular urinalysis (mainly to check on CHO loss)
   (iv) Regular glycosylated haemoglobin or fructosamine estimations (mainly to provide retrospective information on the validity of home glucose monitoring)

   Insulin treatment is best using combined soluble and intermediate-acting insulins morning and evening or intermittent soluble insulin with each meal (three times a day) and an intermediate acting insulin in the evening. Human or highly purified porcine insulins reduce the risk of developing antibodies (which can cross the placenta)

   Maternal health is also monitored carefully, paying particular attention to weight, optic fundi, blood pressure, and renal function

   Fetal welfare should be monitored carefully:
   (i) Offer AFP screening at 16 to 18 weeks
   (ii) Carry out baseline scans to confirm gestational age and exclude major anomalies
   (iii) Continue with serial scans for reduced and excess fetal growth
   (iv) Assess fetal well-being (see p. 45) regularly from 28 weeks

Admission to hospital is indicated if:
(i) Good glucose control cannot be achieved as an outpatient
(ii) Severe H/T and/or proteinuria develop
(iii) Weight gain is excessive
(iv) Renal function deteriorates
(v) Fetal well-being causes concern

3. *Gestational diabetes.* If IGT is discovered during pregnancy carry out blood glucose profile (as above). Treatment is indicated for glucose levels ≥5.8 mmol/l. Dietary control should be attempted initially. If this is not successful then insulin should be prescribed. Management is then as above for established diabetes
4. *Labour and delivery.* When diabetes is well controlled *and pregnancy is uncomplicated* vaginal delivery between 38 and 40 weeks should be anticipated.
During labour close control of blood glucose is achieved by a continuous infusion of soluble insulin (usually 50 u in 50 ml normal saline), and a separate infusion of 5% dextrose with KCl (10 mmol in 500 ml) added. The dextrose and KCl infusion should run at a constant rate (100 ml/h). Regular blood glucose monitoring should be undertaken and the insulin infusion titrated to keep levels between 5 and 7 mmol/l. If a syntocinon infusion is necessary this should be made up using normal saline. Continuous electronic fetal monitoring is advised.

If elective Caesarean section is planned, careful control is necessary before, during and afterwards until the woman can eat and drink normally.

If pre-term labour supervenes, beta-sympathomimetics and steroids are best avoided but, if absolutely necessary, can be covered by appropriate insulin infusions.

5. *Postnatal care.* Insulin sensitivity increases immediately after delivery of the placenta. The required dose of insulin therefore falls quickly and careful monitoring is necessary.

Hypoglycaemia is common in the neonate and must be treated promptly.

Breast feeding is to be encouraged.

Perinatal mortality among diabetic women is now approaching that for other pregnancies (once congenital malformations are excluded), in the best centres.

OTHER ENDOCRINE PROBLEMS

Pituitary

Prolactin secretion increases from the anterior pituitary throughout pregnancy in response to oestrogen stimulation. By term the concentration has increased ten- to twenty-fold. Basal concentrations fall rapidly after delivery but remain above the normal range in lactating women. Suckling induces a prompt release and levels rise five- to ten-fold. Its main role in pregnancy is trophic action on the breast. After delivery it initiates and maintains lactation, and prevents ovulation (a contraceptive function).

Prolactinoma

Expansion of a prolactinoma is unusual during pregnancy. Conservative management is usually appropriate.

1. If being treated with bromocriptine — stop it as soon as pregnancy is diagnosed
2. Check visual fields at 6-week intervals
3. If severe headaches develop or visual fields become impaired admit to hospital. If fetal maturity allows, deliver probably by Caesarean section. As oestrogen levels fall the prolactin level and volume of the prolactinoma will fall. If the fetus is too immature give bromocriptine 5 mg daily doubling each day to 20 mg/day in divided doses or until side-effects prevent further increase
4. If visual fields continue to deteriorate add dexamethasone to reduce intracranial swelling and fetoplacental production of oestrogens and deliver by Caesarean section within 48 hours.

Breast feeding is not contra-indicated in the presence of a prolactinoma.

Thyroid

The main physiological changes in pregnancy are:

1. Renal clearance of iodide doubles in the first trimester and then remains stable. The result is a low plasma iodide. This is only significant when dietary iodine intake is inadequate when goitre can develop
2. The level of thyroid-binding proteins (globulin, pre-albumin and albumin) more than doubles due to an oestrogen effect on the liver. Although total T_3 and T_4 levels rise markedly, the levels of free hormones fall gradually (but remain within normal limits) as pregnancy progresses
3. Basal matabolic rate (BMR) increases by up to 30% by the third trimester. This is necessary because of the requirements of the uterus and fetus (75% of the change) and increased maternal respiratory and cardiac effort (25% of the change)
4. Thyroid stimulating hormone (TSH) levels are unchanged in pregnancy

The pregnant woman is basically euthyroid.

Hyperthyroidism

Complicates about 2 per 1000 pregnancies but it has usually

been diagnosed and treated before pregnancy. The main cause is Graves' disease, but toxic multinodular or solitary nodular goitre may occur. Solitary nodules require careful evaluation because of the risk of malignancy. Fine-needle aspiration is appropriate.

Uncontrolled hyperthyroidism is associated with increased risk of IUGR, pre-term labour and fetal and neonatal death. The most frequent cause is an auto-antibody (long-acting thyroid stimulator [LATS]) which crosses the placenta. It may cause neonatal hyperthyroidism which has a high mortality rate (up to 25% of cases).

Signs and symptoms

The symptoms overlap with those of normal pregnancy, and palpable thyroid enlargement may be physiological in pregnancy. Biochemical diagnosis is essential.

Diagnosis: free T_3 raised; free T_4 raised or normal; TSH suppressed.

Treatment: carbimazole or propylthiouracil with thyroxine supplement. These drugs cross the placenta and can therefore affect the fetal thyroid. However, the balance of risk is in their favour. Propranolol may be used to control serious peripheral effects of thyrotoxicosis. When control is achieved the drugs can be reduced gradually. Breastfeeding is not necessarily contra-indicated.

Sub-total thyroidectomy may be indicated if a large goitre is causing obstruction, drugs fail to control the symptoms, or there are toxic reactions to drugs.

Babies born to thyrotoxic mothers should be screened for hypothyroidism.

Hypothyroidism

Myxoedema rarely presents in pregnancy because sufferers tend to be infertile.

Treated hypothyroidism due to auto-immune disease or following partial thyroidectomy is not uncommon (about 9 per 1000 pregnancies).

Untreated hypothyroidism in early pregnancy has a high fetal wastage or can lead to mental retardation, deafness and cerebral palsy. Later in pregnancy cretinism results. The main causes of primary hypothyroidism are idiopathic, Hashimoto's thyroiditis and post-ablative.

Signs and symptoms

Cold intolerance, changes in skin or hair texture; delayed reflexes, bradycardia. A goitre may be present.

Diagnosis: free T_4 reduced; TSH high.

These can also be used to test adequacy of replacement therapy.

Treatment: thyroxine replacement. Breast-feeding is not contra-indicated. If mother has previously had thyrotoxicosis check for neonatal thyrotoxicosis. If she has had auto-immune thyroiditis check baby for hypothyroidism.

Postpartum thyroiditis

This is said to occur in 5 to 9% of pregnancies and is generally unrecognised. It presents with fatigue, palpitations or other features of mild hyperthyroidism 2 to 4 months postpartum, and is often confused with 'postpartum blues'. It is commonly associated with HLA DR3, 4 or 5. Up to 25% of affected women will have a first-degree relative with a history of thyroid disease. Such women should be screened for thyroid antibodies at booking.

Diagnosis: T_3 and T_4 levels are raised. Radioactive iodine uptake is low. Thyroid antimicrosomal antibodies are present.

Treatment: it is usually a self-limiting condition, but hypothyroidism may persist in a small minority. In the thyrotoxic phase beta-blocking agents may be used. In the hypothyroid phase thyroxine can be given for 4 to 6 months.

Adrenal cortex

Among the physiological changes which occur in pregnancy are:

1. Aldosterone levels rise within days of conception due to an increase in angiotensin II. This reaction is necessary in pregnancy to conserve sodium
2. Plasma cortisol levels, both bound and free, are elevated with loss of the normal diurnal variation. This increase is due to a slight rise in ACTH as a result of placental secretion
3. Deoxycorticosterone (DOC) shows the largest increase of all adrenal steroids, starting by eight weeks' gestation. DOC is not suppressible by dexamethasone during pregnancy. It may be intimately involved with parturition
4. Plasma testosterone rises secondary to the rise in sex hormone-binding globulin, although it is likely that unbound testosterone is unchanged

Addison's disease (Primary hypoadrenalism)

This is a rare complication of pregnancy. If diagnosed and treated before pregnancy, corticosteroid therapy must continue. Additional supplementation will be necessary at times of stress (e.g. labour) or if any infection occurs.

The clinical manifestations of previously undiagnosed Addison's disease (including pigmentation) are common in normal pregnancy. A suspected diagnosis can be confirmed by low urine or plasma cortisol levels which do not respond to ACTH. The stress of labour and delivery can precipitate an acute crisis among the features of which are nausea, vomiting, diarrhoea, abdominal (usually flank) pain, and debility. The woman is febrile and hypotensive. It is accompanied by low sodium, high potassium and increased urea levels with a metabolic acidosis. A refractory hypoglycaemia may occur.

Emergency treatment

1. Hydrocortisone (but not mineralocorticoids) by i.v. infusion
2. Electrolyte replacement and correction of acidosis as necessary
3. Vigorous treatment of any infection
4. Monitor urine output carefully

Cushing's syndrome

This is a rare but serious condition in pregnancy. Fetal loss is common and there is a significant risk to the mother's life. The main causes are pituitary adenoma, and adrenocortical adenoma or carcinoma. The presentation is as in the non-pregnant (see *Aids to Postgraduate Medicine*). Firm diagnosis is so important that CT scanning of adrenals and pituitary are indicated. Management depends on the stage in pregnancy when the condition is diagnosed:

First trimester — termination of pregnancy must be considered with definitive treatment thereafter

Second trimester — miscarriage is likely. Metyrapone therapy and/or surgery must be considered

Third trimester — (a) early: metyrapone therapy until fetus is mature enough to be delivered; (b) late: prompt delivery and definitive treatment. Caesarean section should be covered by metyrapone and glucocorticoid therapy

Adrenal medulla — phaeochromocytoma

The catecholamines adrenaline and noradrenaline do not change in pregnancy. This tumour rarely complicates pregnancy, but the consequences for the mothers are serious if it goes undetected. Only about half the cases are diagnosed antenatally.
Patients may present with sustained or paroxysmal hypertension. The other classical symptoms of headache, palpitations and excess sweating may not occur in pregnancy. It is a cause of sudden collapse in pregnancy, labour or the puerperium. It should be excluded when severe or intermittent hypertension occurs (particularly in early pregnancy); in the presence of above 'classical' symptoms; in women with a family history of phaeochromocytoma or associated syndromes, e.g. neurofibromatosis or multiple endocrine neoplasia.
Diagnosis: estimation of catecholamines in a properly collected 24-hour urine sample. Ultrasound may detect a suprarenal mass. CT scan or MRI are useful for further localisation.
Treatment: alpha adrenergic blockade using phenoxybenzamine.

Control may take 10 to 14 days. Beta adrenergic blockage using Propanolol may be necessary to treat tachyarrhythmias. Alpha blockade must be achieved first. Before 23 weeks' gestation the tumour should be removed. From 24 weeks' gestation the pregnant uterus makes this technically difficult. Surgical removal can be delayed until fetal maturity is adequate as long as alpha blockade is achieved. Removal is best combined with elective Caesarean section. Specialist anaesthesia is required, and initial postoperative management must be in an intensive care unit.

IMMUNOLOGICAL DISORDERS

For a description of the immune system and its function see Suggested further reading.

The major factors protecting the semi-allogeneic (foreign) fetus and placenta from maternal immune attack are:

1. The absence of class I (HLA A,B,C) and class II (HLA DP, DQ, DR) major histocompatibility complex (MHC) antigens from villous trophoblast
2. The presence on extravillous trophoblast of non-classical MHC antigens to which T cells cannot respond
3. Protective responses may occur to minor trophoblast antigens
4. Local immune responses may be suppressed by non-specific suppressor cells and other factors in the maternal decidua

The placenta acts as a barrier to the passage of maternal cells to the fetus. IgG, but not IgM, is actively transported. This provides passive immunity to the fetus but can also cause pathology, e.g. Rhesus haemolytic disease, and allo-immune thrombocytopaenia.

Immune thrombocytopaenia

Platelet mass and turnover increase in pregnancy. The count may fall slightly in normal pregnancy. Thrombocytopaenia is defined as a platelet count below $100 \times 10^9 \, l^{-1}$.

Auto-immune (or idiopathic) thrombocytopaenia (ITP)

IgG antiplatelet auto-antibodies bind to platelet-specific antigens and cause them to be sequestered in the spleen. ITP occurs more commonly in women than in men, with a peak incidence at the height of the reproductive years. It affects about 1 per 1000 pregnancies.

Maternal risks have been overstated. The major hazard is postpartum haemorrhage with an incidence of over 30% if platelet count is below $100 \times 10^9 \, l^{-1}$.

Fetal risk. The IgG antiplatelet antibodies cross the placenta, but maternal platelet count is a poor predictor of fetal/neonatal thrombocytopaenia. The principal fetal risk is *intracranial haemorrhage* (ICH) but this has been overstated. There is no

evidence that elective Caesarean section reduces the risk, but it is indicated in the pre-term infant and for breech presentation.
Investigation of mother with ITP. If platelet count $\geq 100 \times 10^9\ l^{-1}$ check it at booking, 28, and 34 weeks, and at onset of labour. If count $< 50 \times 10^9\ l^{-1}$, or if there is haemorrhage, exclude other causes — e.g. clotting disorder, pre-eclampsia. The value of measuring platelet auto-antibodies is not proven.
Investigation of fetus. Antenatal ultrasound can help to exclude ICH in utero. *Fetal scalp sampling* in labour is not helpful. *Cordocentesis* will give an accurate picture of the fetal state but its morbidity does not justify its use except under exceptional circumstances.
Treatment: *corticosteroids* — if maternal platelet count $< 50 \times 10^9\ l^{-1}$. *Immunoglobulin* infusion is best restricted to steroid resistant cases. *Platelet transfusions* give only short-lived benefit. They can be used to cover delivery if platelet count is $< 30 \times 10^9\ l^{-1}$. *Plasmaphoresis* may be used when other medical management has failed. *Splenectomy* is justified only if serious haemorrhage has failed to respond to conservative treatment, with platelet count $< 30 \times 10^9\ l^{-1}$.

A normal platelet count in a woman who has had a splenectomy does not mean that the fetus is unaffected.

Allo-immune thrombocytopaenia
This is analogous to Rhesus disease. Maternal platelets are normal but the mother may develop antibodies against fetal platelet antigens, usually $P1A_1$ (or Zw^a). The incidence may be as high as 1–2 per 1000 pregnancies. The first pregnancy is affected in up to 50% of cases. Lack of $P1A_1$ antigen in the mother could be the basis for a screening test. The fetus is at significant risk of ICH. Cordocentesis is justified for the fetus at risk, and fetal immunoglobulin or platelets can be given if indicated. Elective Caesarean section is indicated if the fetal platelet count is $< 50 \times 10^9\ l^{-1}$.

Systemic lupus erythematosus (SLE)
SLE is a multisystem disease of unknown aetiology that tends to occur in women of reproductive age. The diagnosis rests on the presence of criteria suggested by the American Rheumatism Association (see Tan et al, in Suggested further reading). The most helpful serological tests are anti-nuclear factor and anti-DNA antibodies.

Pregnancy has no specific effects on SLE except for an increased risk of exacerbation during the puerperium. Women with SLE in pregnancy have an increased risk of:

1. First-trimester pregnancy loss
2. Lupus nephritis

3. Hypertension in pregnancy
4. Transient neonatal SLE — permanent congenital heart block may occur in association with anti-Ro antibodies. A seemingly healthy woman delivering a baby with CHB should be observed for the development of SLE.

Management during pregnancy
Close antenatal supervision is necessary with particular attention to serial measurements of blood pressure, renal function and fetal growth.

The mainstay of treatment is maternal corticosteroid therapy but azathioprine may be needed in some circumstances.

The timing of delivery depends on the severity of the condition, and deteriorating renal function may be an indication for early delivery.

If the fetus has congenital heart block then Caesarean section is warranted.

Lupus anticoagulant (LA) or inhibitor
A circulating anti-cardiolipin antibody which acts on the clotting cascade. All phospholipid-dependent coagulation tests, e.g. activated partial thromboplastin time (APTT) and kaolin clotting time (KCT), tend to be prolonged even after the addition of normal plasma. It is associated with a high prevalence of maternal thrombosis and fetal loss. It is not specific to SLE and may be found in any woman with a history of unexplained fetal loss at any gestational age.

Corticosteroids and low-dose aspirin have been used successfully to treat affected women.

Myasthenia gravis
This is a rare auto-immune condition with a peak incidence between 20 and 30 years of age. It produces rapid fatigue and weakness of voluntary muscles. It is frequently associated with a thymoma or thymic lymphoid hyperplasia. Pregnancy does not worsen the disease but exacerbations can occur (most frequently in the puerperium) in up to 30% of women.

The antibody can cross the placenta and cause a transient (or rarely permanent) effect on fetal voluntary muscles.

Treatment is with anticholinesterase drugs such as neostigmine (with atropine) or pyridostigmine. Corticosteroids or ACTH may also be effective. Among the drugs which can exacerbate it are sedatives, tranquillisers, analgesics and narcotics. General anaesthesia requiring muscle relaxation can result in prolonged paralysis of voluntary muscles. Labour may be shorter than usual but the effort of the second stage can be tiring. Elective forceps delivery is usually indicated.

RHESUS ISO-IMMUNISATION

The Rh factor

Each Rh gene is made up of three components from three allelomorphic pairs — C or c̄, D or d, E or e. Each parent passes on either the first or second half of his/her full genotype, e.g. CDe/c̄de parents hand on their CDe or c̄de.

All Rh-negative people have 'd' in each half of the genotype. Where 'D' occurs in both halves of the genotype a parent is homozygous and passes on only the Rh-D-positive gene.

Clinically significant rhesus iso-immunisation is usually against the D antigen. Anti-c̄ or anti-Kell antibodies may also cause problems.

Sensitisation

Usually occurs at parturition due to feto-maternal haemorrhage. Other causes of transplacental haemorrhage include abortion (spontaneous or induced), abruptio placentae, amniocentesis and external cephalic version.

Prevention

Anti-D immunoglobulin 500 i.u. (100 μg) can eliminate up to 4.0 ml of Rh-D-positive blood from the maternal circulation. It should be given in this dose to all Rh-D-negative women delivering an Rh-D-positive infant from 20 weeks' gestation or after a severe placental abruption. It must be given within 60 hours of the event. If a Kleihauer test demonstrates a feto-maternal transfusion (FMT) of >4.0 ml additional anti-D must be given.

250 i.u. (50 μg) should be given to Rh-D-negative women as soon as possible after a potentially sensitising event. Any FMT > 2.0 ml requires additional anti-D.

The continued occurrence of Rh iso-immunisation is due to:

(i) Failure to give any or enough anti-D when indicated

(ii) Sensitisation during a first pregnancy in the absence of complications. This may occur in up to 2% of Rh-D negative primigravidae. The routine injection of anti-D 500 i.u. at 28 and 34 weeks would reduce Rh-D sensitisation in primigravidae by a factor of 8.

Detection

In unsensitised women check for Rh antibodies at booking, 28, 32 and 36 weeks.

Prediction of severity

1. Obstetric history

It tends to become more severe in successive pregnancies. If at least one child has died from rhesus haemolytic disease the chance of this pregnancy ending successfully is less than 50%.

2. Husband's genotype
About 75% of the fathers of affected children are homozygous ($R_1 R_1$).

3. Maternal antibody levels
Once antibodies are detected they must be measured at least monthly thereafter. Serum antibody protein levels are of greater predictive value than antibody titres. A rapid increase suggests that acute haemolysis will be occurring in the fetus and amniotic fluid analysis is necessary.

4. Amniotic fluid analysis
Maternal IgG crosses the placenta and will cause a fetal haemolytic anaemia. Amniotic fluid bilirubin concentrations correlate well with the severity of the haemolysis.

Spectrophotometry at an optical density (OD) of 450 nm shows a peak directly proportional to the quantity of bilirubin. If a previous pregnancy has been complicated by Rh-isoimmunisation, the first amniocentesis should be 10 weeks before the earliest previous intrauterine transfusion, intrauterine death or delivery of fatally or severely affected infant, but not before 20 weeks, gestation.

The second should be 3 to 4 weeks later. The necessity for, and interval between, subsequent amniocenteses are determined by bilirubin levels.

5. Fetal blood sampling
Fetal blood sampling under ultrasound guidance can be used to check fetal haematocrit. It is indicated in patients at risk of severe early disease or if amniotic fluid analysis in later second and third trimesters suggests that the baby is severely affected.

Intrauterine transfusion
If the fetus is severely affected between 24 and 31 weeks' gestation direct intravascular fetal blood transfusion (IVT) can be carried out under ultrasound guidance; transfusions can be repeated fortnightly. It is particularly useful if hydrops is present, but should be carried out only in specialised centres. Intraperitoneal transfusion can be used in conjunction with IVT in the absence of hydrops.

Testing the baby at birth
Cord blood is taken routinely from the babies of all Rh-D-negative mothers for Hb and film, Coombs' test and bilirubin levels.

RESPIRATORY DISEASES

1. Bronchial asthma

Pregnancy has no consistent effect on asthma, and cases should be managed medically in the normal manner using sympathomimetic bronchodilators (e.g. salbutamol or orciprenaline) or disodium cromoglycate. If steroids are used, or have been recently, cover labour (for anaesthesia) with hydrocortisone (inhaled steroids do not need parenteral cover during labour).

Status asthmaticus is treated by steroids in high doses, bronchodilators and artificial ventilation, if necessary.

2. Pulmonary tuberculosis

If the diagnosis is made during pregnancy treat with isoniazid and PAS or ethambutol. Breast-feeding is contra-indicated if the patient has sputum-positive TB. The infant requires BCG vaccination and should be separated from the mother only if she has open TB and until Mantoux conversion.

EPILEPSY

Pre-pregnancy counselling is important for women with epilepsy in order to:

1. Check their anticonvulsant therapy for need, safety and dosage
2. Allay their many fears about pregnancy and nursing a small baby

The risk of an epileptic mother having an epileptic baby is about 1:40. Pregnancy does not provoke epilepsy in mothers but the frequency of seizures may increase because anticonvulsants are cleared more quickly.

Teratogenicity of anticonvulsants

The incidence of congenital malformations is increased two to three-fold in infants of women on anticonvulsants. No one drug is free of risk, but phenytoin (alone or in combination) is implicated most frequently. Among the problems are:

1. Cleft lip and/or palate (increased ten-fold)
2. Congenital heart defect (increased four-fold)
3. Hypoplasia of terminal phalanges of fingers
4. Possible characteristic facial appearance: wide-spaced eyes, low posterior hair line, short neck, prominent brow and trigoncephaly
5. Retarded growth, delayed development and, occasionally, mental retardation

Sodium valproate is associated with fetal spina bifida in about 1% of 'at risk' pregnancies.

Management
Prescribe anticonvulsants in doses sufficient to prevent convulsions. Single-drug therapy should be aimed for if possible. Vitamin K should be given to all neonates (1 mg i.m.). Breast-feeding is not contra-indicated.

Status epilepticus is best treated with intravenous diazepam. The airway must be kept patent and oxygen administered.

DISEASES OF LIVER AND ALIMENTARY TRACT

Jaundice — incidence approximately 1:1500 pregnancies.

Jaundice caused by pregnancy

Intrahepatic cholestasis (20% of cases)
The patient has pruritus in the second half of pregnancy (some never become jaundiced). Bilirubin and transaminases are slightly elevated.

It is associated with some increased risk of pre-term labour, fetal distress and perinatal death. It clears up after delivery and does not proceed to chronic liver disease. It tends to recur in subsequent pregnancies and may also occur in association with oestrogen-containing oral contraceptives.

Cholestyramine will reduce itching but is very unpleasant to take. Parenteral vitamin K is required if jaundice causes prolongation of the prothrombin time.

Jaundice complicating pre-eclampsia — see p. 62

Intercurrent jaundice in pregnancy

Viral hepatitis (40% of cases)
Due either to hepatitis B (long incubation, serum hepatitis) or hepatitis A (short incubation, infective hepatitis). Hepatitis B is discussed on p. 101.

Cholelithiasis (6% of cases)
Modern ultrasound or transhepatic cholangiography may be useful in confirming the diagnosis.

Cholecystectomy can be carried out in pregnancy, preferably in the second trimester.

Drug toxicity — see Haemolysis

Haemolysis
These are rare causes, but should be considered.

Pre-existing liver disease
Pregnancy is uncommon in the presence of cirrhosis due, for example, to active chronic hepatitis, or primary biliary cirrhosis.

The prognosis is good for mother and baby in familial non-haemolytic jaundice, e.g. Gilbert's and the Dubin-Johnson syndromes. Pregnancy may increase jaundice in the latter.

Gastric reflux and hiatus hernia
The lower oesophagel sphincter relaxes under the influence of pregnancy hormones. Reflux of acid gastric contents leads to *heartburn*. This can also be due to a 'sliding' *hiatus hernia*.

Management
Frequent small meals; advise patient to avoid lying flat; simple antacids. If no relief is obtained 'floating' antacids, or metoclopramide, can be tried. Dilute hydrochloric acid has also proved successful.

Peptic ulceration
Peptic ulcers tend to improve in pregnancy. H_2-receptor antagonists may be necessary in some cases but their long-term use is not recommended. Perforation of a peptic ulcer should be managed surgically as in the non-pregnant patient.

Coeliac disease
Coeliac disease may present in pregnancy as a folate deficiency anaemia.

If untreated it may be associated with an increased risk of abortion or intrauterine growth retardation. It is successfully treated by a gluten-free diet and vitamin supplements.

Ulcerative colitis
Ulcerative colitis does not affect pregnancy adversely.

Pregnancy does not increase the chance of relapse of quiescent colitis, but if the colitis arises *de novo* in pregnancy or the puerperium it carries a poor prognosis. Treatment can continue during pregnancy with rectal and systemic steroids and/or sulphasalazine.

In the presence of an ileostomy most pregnancies proceed to normal vaginal delivery.

Crohn's disease
There may be a small adverse effect on fetal outcome due to the disease. The condition itself is usually unaffected by pregnancy.

Deterioration is most likely in the puerperium. It should be managed in the same manner as in the non-pregnant.

PSYCHIATRIC DISORDERS

Post-partum 'blues'
This is not an illness but rather a transient mild disturbance characterised by

weeping	feelings of helplessness
irritability	sensitivity to criticism
variation in mood	poor sleep

It occurs in at least 50% of postpartum women, usually develops around the third day, and may last for a few hours or days.

Treatment is by psychological support and reassurance.

Depressive illness
Often brought on by psycho-social stress, and there may be a previous psychiatric history. Peak incidence is 3 months postpartum. Characterised by tiredness, lethargy, irritability and anxiety which may be more prominent than depression.

Treatment is by psychological and practical support and antidepressant drugs as necessary.

Puerperal psychosis
This presents either as an affective disorder with depression or hypomania, or schizophrenia with delusions and hallucinations. It often begins within 4 days of delivery. The incidence is about 2 per 1000 live births.

A psychiatrist must be consulted because there is risk of suicide and harm to or neglect of the baby.

There is an increased risk of psychotic illness in the future, including during further pregnancies.

Mono-amine oxidase inhibitors are best avoided in pregnancy, but withdrawal must be gradual.

Drug abuse
The social outlook for the baby is very poor. Drug abusers are poor antenatal clinic attenders and may present for the first time in labour. Examine arms for scars, tattoo marks and thrombophlebitis.

Opiates
Intravenous abuse of heroin or methadone (Physeptone) with dirty syringes carries among its risks hepatitis B and HIV infections, septicaemia, syphilis and rhesus sensitisation.

Give pethidine or methadone during labour.

Sudden withdrawal can cause fetal death, so gradual weaning is necessary.

The infant must not be given opiate antagonists (e.g. nalorphine).

THROMBO-EMBOLISM

Coagulation and fibrinolysis during normal pregnancy
Factors VII, VIII, IX and X are increased from the beginning of the second trimester. The most marked increase is in plasma

fibrinogen. This results in a relative hypercoagulable state ready to cope with placental separation at delivery. Plasma fibrinolytic activity is decreased and returns to normal within 15 minutes of delivery of the placenta. Plasmin inhibitors (e.g. $alpha_2$ macroglobulin and $alpha_1$ antitrypsin) increase substantially.
Superficial thrombo-phlebitis does not carry a significant risk of thrombo-embolism unless it extends to the deep veins.
Deep vein thrombosis (DVT). Signs: oedema, local tenderness, increase in diameter of the leg, a positive Homan's sign. Most cases are less obvious and some are silent.

Diagnosis

(i) Venography
(ii) Ultrasonic detection of venous patency is inadequate
(iii) Radioactive fibrinogen uptake is contra-indicated

The main complications are pulmonary embolism and chronic vascular insufficiency.

Pulmonary embolism

There may be no prior clinical evidence of DVT. It is one of the commonest causes of maternal death.

Factors associated with increased risk

Increasing age and parity
Obesity
Confinement to bed
Suppression of lactation with oestrogens
Caesarean section (particularly in pre-eclamptic women)
Blood groups other than O
Sickle-cell disease

Signs and symptoms

Pleuritic pain, haemoptysis, dyspnoea and varying degrees of shock.

Consider also if there is no other obvious explanation for tachycardia, pyrexia or bronchospasm.

Investigation

1. Chest X-ray may be helpful but can be totally normal
2. ECG — usually normal except when the embolus is large and has produced acute cor pulmonale. Even these changes may be obscured by the usual ECG changes which occur in pregnancy
3. Ventilation — perfusion isotope lung scan
4. Pulmonary angiography may need to be considered

Management of DVT and pulmonary embolism

Acute therapy
Intravenous calcium heparin 40 000 units daily (in saline by infusion pump) for at least 48 hours. Its action is to inhibit thrombin and factors IX, X, XI and XII.

Long-term therapy
Heparin can be continued subcutaneously or Warfarin can be substituted.

1. *Subcutaneous heparin* inhibits activated factor X without prolonging the clotting time.
   The initial dose is 10 000 units twice daily. This may be reduced to 5000 units twice daily depending on plasma heparin levels which should be kept between 0.2 and 0.6 units/ml.
   This level does not add to the risk of haemorrhage even at Caesarean section. It should be continued for at least 6 weeks postpartum (or Warfarin be substituted after delivery). Heparin-induced maternal osteoporosis can occur after long-term therapy in pregnancy
2. *Warfarin* inhibits the synthesis of vitamin K-dependent clotting factors (II, VII, IX and X).
   It is best avoided in the first trimester because of a slight risk of embryopathy. Meticulous control is vital — keep prothrombin time to 2 to 2.5 times the clotting time for a normal control plasma. Its anticoagulant effect cannot be reversed rapidly, therefore stop Warfarin and change to heparin at 36 weeks' gestation.
   If labour supervenes while the patient is taking Warfarin it can be counteracted with fresh frozen plasma and vitamin K1. Warfarin crosses the placenta but not into the breast milk to any significant extent. Breast-feeding is not contra-indicated. It should be continued for 6 weeks after delivery

Prophylaxis of thrombo-embolism (TE)

The risk of recurrence in a woman with a past history of thrombo-embolism occurring in pregnancy or while on 'the pill' is said to be about 12%, but the majority of these occur postnatally. The following is a guide to policy:

1. History of one episode in the past — give infusion of 500–1000 ml of dextran 70 during labour and continue with subcutaneous heparin or Warfarin for 6 weeks
2. If the history of TE is equivocal or dubious, anticoagulants are probably not indicated
3. Anticoagulation is necessary throughout pregnancy for those at high risk of recurrence of TE, e.g. patients with:

(i) History of multiple episodes
(ii) Antithrombin III deficiency
4. Treat women with history of TE who are admitted to hospital for bed rest
5. Consider treatment in the puerperium for the obese grande multipara with varicose veins, or who has had an operative delivery

MALIGNANT DISEASE AND PREGNANCY

Pregnancy does not usually adversely affect the course of malignant disease. The poor prognosis of pregnant women with cervical cancer is more likely to be due to the aggressiveness of the tumour in women in that age group than to the pregnancy itself.

The disease can effect the pregnancy and fetus by:
1. Transplacental transmission of tumour cells — this occurs only very rarely
2. Maternal effects, e.g. increased risk of infection in leukaemia, or cachexia
3. Increased maternal mortality
4. The effects of therapy, e.g. anomalies and IUGR

Termination of pregnancy is not of itself therapeutic but it may be inevitable in some cases, either before or as a consequence of chemo- or radio-therapy.

Cervical cancer and CIN

Perform a cervical smear at the booking antenatal clinic if the woman has never had one before or not within the past 5 years. If the smear is abnormal carry out colposcopy — colposcopically-directed biopsies can be taken safely in pregnancy.

Cervical intra-epithelial neoplasia (CIN) should be serially observed for the remainder of pregnancy and dealt with definitively at the end of the puerperium.

Invasive carcinoma of the cervix poses several clinical problems in pregnancy.
1. If discovered under 22 weeks' gestation advise termination (by hysterotomy) followed by definitive treatment (see p. 263)
2. Between 22 and 26 weeks it may be justifiable to await fetal viability before ending the pregnancy
3. Thereafter delivery should be effected in consultation with a neonatal paediatrician and the woman herself

Vaginal delivery is contra-indicated. Whatever the management, the prognosis is poor.

Ovarian cancer

Ovarian tumours of all varieties are said to complicate 1 in 1000 pregnancies, although only 1 in 20 are malignant. The frequency of tumour types is as in the non-pregnant woman (see p. 278)

Ultrasound is useful for detection of ovarian swellings.

Management

Treat as in the non-pregnant woman (see p. 284). The prognosis seems to be better for ovarian cancer in pregnancy with a 5-year survival rate of up to 75% compared to an overall 25%. This reflects the nature of the tumours in this age group.

Breast cancer

This is the commonest malignant tumour to affect women. About 2% of women under 45 years of age who have the disease are pregnant at the time of diagnosis.

Lymph node involvement seems to be increased in pregnancy. Prognosis may, therefore, be poorer.

Antenatal and post-natal examination of the breasts should be routine.

Management

1. In the first half of pregnancy treatment should be as for the non-pregnant woman; if chemotherapy is necessary termination is advisable
2. In the second half of pregnancy delivery should be effected if the fetus is viable; treatment can then begin

   It may be justifiable to delay treatment for a short time to await fetal viability in some cases
3. Breast-feeding is probably contra-indicated.

Further pregnancies can be embarked on if desired after a post-treatment interval of 2 years.

Hodgkin's disease

This affects about 1 in 6000 pregnant women.

Management

1. In the first half of pregnancy radiotherapy can be carried out with shielding of the uterus and ovaries
2. In later pregnancy chemo- and radio-therapy can sometimes be delayed until after delivery

Melanoma

Pregnancy appears to have no significant influence on survival. Pregnancy is probably best avoided for three years following excision because most recurrences occur within that time. Management of a melanoma found in pregnancy is as for the non-pregnant woman. Transplacental spread to the fetus is exceedingly rare.

SUGGESTED FURTHER READING

Brudenell M, Wilds P L 1984 Medical and surgical problem in obstetrics. Wright, Bristol

de Swiet M (ed) 1984 Medical disorders in obstetrics practice. Blackwell, Oxford

Greer I A 1989 Thromboembolic problem in pregnancy. Fetal Medicine Review 1: 79–103

Howie P W 1986 Anticoagulants in pregnancy. In: Beeley L, Stirrat G M (eds) Prescribing in pregnancy. Clinics in obstetrics and gynaecology. Saunders, Eastbourne, Vol 13, No. 2,

Kumar R 1985 Pregnancy, childbirth and mental illness. In: Studd J (ed) Progress in obstetrics and gynaecology. Churchill Livingstone, Edinburgh, Vol 5, p. 134

Lindheimer M D, Barron W M (eds) 1985 Medical disorders during pregnancy. Clinics in perinatology. Saunders, Philadelphia, Vol 12, No. 3

Shepherd J H 1984 Cancer in pregnancy. In: Studd J (ed) Progress in obstetrics and gynaecology. Churchill Livingstone, Edinburgh, Vol 4, p. 219

Tan E M et al 1982 The 1982 revised criteria for the classification of systemic lupus erythematosus. Arthritis and Rheumatism, 25, 1271–7

Tuck S M 1984 Sickle cell disease and pregnancy. In: Chamberlain G (ed) Contemporary obstetrics. Butterworth, London, p. 57

Turnbull A, Chamberlain G 1989 Obstetrics. Churchill Livingstone, Edinburgh

Vaughan N J A, Oakley N W 1986 Treatment of diabetes in pregnancy. In: Beeley L, Stirrat G M (eds) Prescribing in pregnancy. Clinics in obstetrics and gynaecology. Saunders, Eastbourne, Vol 13, No. 2,

Maternal and fetal infections

SEXUALLY TRANSMITTED DISEASES

Infections caused by *Candida albicans, Trichomonas vaginalis* and *Neisseria gonorrhoeae* are included within the general discussion on STDs (p. 215).

Treponemal infections

Syphilis, yaws and pinta are all caused by treponemes which are indistinguishable morphologically and serologically. Clinically apparent syphilis is rare in pregnancy but failure to diagnose it can have severe long-term effects on mother and child. Routine antenatal screening is therefore still indicated and cost effective.

Syphilis is still rife in developing countries.

Screening for syphilis

Blood is taken at booking for VDRL (Venereal Disease Reference Laboratory) or RPR (Reiter protein reagin) and TPHA (*Treponema pallidum* haemagglutination) test.

Further action is necessary if screening tests are positive, there is a history of contact or there is clinical evidence of syphilis. More specific tests can then be carried out:

(i) FTA[abs] (fluorescent treponemal antibody-absorbed) the most sensitive test for syphilis. FTA[abs] IgM indicates recent infection but may give a transient false-positive reaction with herpes infections.

(ii) TPI (*Treponema pallidum* immobilisation) — the most specific test but less sensitive than FTA[abs] or TPHA.

Biological false-positive reactions (BFPR) are much commoner than true infections and may occur spontaneously in pregnancy, and after blood transfusion or recent vaccination as well as many other conditions (e.g. SLE). FTA[abs] and TPI are negative in BFPR detected by other tests.

Treatment of syphilis

Use penicillin unless the patient is allergic. With a history of mild (non-anaphylactic) allergy use cephaloridine.

With severe (anaphylactic) allergies use erythromycin. It may be best to re-treat women in subsequent pregnancies.

Discuss appropriate drug and dose with microbiologist.

Congenital syphilis
Syphilis can have serious effects on every organ and system in the developing fetus and early maternal syphilis carries a high rate of fetal infection. Adequate treatment of the mother before 16 weeks of pregnancy will prevent infection in virtually all cases. Treatment after this time will still be effective in most cases.

Herpes simplex virus (HSV)
HSV Type 2 causes 70% of herpetic genital-tract infections. Small vulval or vaginal vesicles may become painful ulcers. Diagnosis is by culture in special viral culture medium. Acyclovir cream reduces the duration of signs and symptoms.

Routine screening of all pregnant women is not recommended.

The fetus has no intrinsic immunity to the virus and no passive immunity during a primary maternal infection. Transmission of herpes infection from mother to the fetus/baby is high (40%) after vaginal delivery in primary maternal infection but low (3%) if infection is recurrent. The following policy is therefore suggested:

1. *Primary infection with active genital lesions*
   (i) Delivery by Caesarean section if labour occurs and if membranes intact, or within 4 hours of membrane rupture. Take viral swabs from baby
   (ii) If more than 4 hours since membrane rupture allow vaginal delivery because Caesarean section will not reduce risk of neonatal infection. Take viral swabs from baby and treat him/her with acyclovir
2. *Secondary infection with active genital lesions*
   Although the perceived risk of neonatal infection is much less its extent is not fully known. The above policy tends to be adopted in the absence of good evidence to the contrary
3. *Asymptomatic viral shedding*
   Allow vaginal delivery and take viral swabs from infant. In the United States it has been shown that a policy of weekly viral cultures in later pregnancy and delivery by Caesarean section for those with positive culture would prevent two cases of neonatal herpes, cause two maternal deaths and cost $37 million

Inoculation risk (IR) women
The following have an increased likelihood of carrying hepatitis B virus, HIV or other agents spread by inoculation:

1. Those with known or suspected AIDS or ARC

2. Those who are HIV antibody positive
3. Those who are or have recently been HBsAg positive/anti HBe negative
4. Those with a history of acute hepatitis in past 6 weeks*
5. Those with chronic active hepatitis or cirrhosis*
6. Those whose childhood was spent outside Northern Europe, North America, Australia or New Zealand**
7. Those who have visited Central Africa in past 5 years**
8. Those with conditions treated using blood products**
9. Sexual partners of HIV risk men**
10. Intravenous drug abusers

Babies of HIV-positive mothers are also included.

All blood or other body fluids being sent to laboratories from IR women must be clearly identified. All personnel dealing with IR women should be immunised against Hep. B.

HIV infection

For detailed discussion see Suggested further reading. The prevalence of HIV infection is unknown, and accurate data are urgently required. Of known infected women in the UK 80% contracted the virus heterosexually or from infected blood products. The largest increase in numbers and proportion of acquired immunodeficiency syndrome (AIDS) is in the heterosexual transmission group.

Screening

Testing without consent is deemed unethical. Testing of 'high-risk' women, e.g. i.v. drug users, prostitutes, and those from Central Africa assumes that the leading questions are answered truthfully and that consent is given. Special precautions should still be taken in handling blood and other body fluids from women at 'high risk' who refuse HIV testing.

Management of HIV-positive pregnant women

Pregnancy and HIV infection probably do not have any adverse effect on each other. There is a 3 out of 4 chance that the baby will be unaffected. Screen for other STDs and other infectious diseases (e.g. toxoplasmosis, CMV, tuberculosis). If symptoms or signs suggesting AIDS or AIDS-related complex (ARC) develop seek help of experts. Sensitive and sympathetic counselling is vital.

Hepatitis B virus

Its presence is demonstrated by testing for its surface antigen HBsAg. A positive result suggests that hepatitis is, or has

*Can be excluded if found to be HBsAg-negative *HBsAg and anti-HBe positive*

**Can be excluded if HIV-negative and more than 1 year since last exposure

recently been, present, or that the woman is a carrier. Carriers who have antibodies to the *e* antigen of the virus (anti-HBe-positive) are not infectious but should not be blood donors.

Babies of HBsAg-positive/HBe-negative women should be given Hep. B gamma globulin and vaccine.

Care of IR women in labour and postnatally

1. Make sure there is a well defined policy for caring for all inoculation-risk (IR) patients including those HIV positive.
2. It is advised that those looking after IR women in labour should:
   (i) Wear adequate eye protection, protective clothing and double gloves, particularly for operative delivery
   (ii) Avoid needle stick injuries
   (iii) Handle body fluids with care and dispose of soiled garments as per above policy
   (iv) Sterilise instruments by autoclave
3. Try to avoid use of fetal scalp clip and sampling to minimise risk of transmission to neonate
4. Warn paediatricians of forthcoming delivery
5. Avoid mouth-operated suction devices

Postnatal care

A single room is preferable, but other women and babies in a shared room are not at increased risk. Dispose of towels, linen, etc. safely. Breast-feeding is probably not advised on the grounds that the viruses can be found in breast milk.

These policies must be continually re-evaluated in the light of new information. Resources must be made available to reduce the hazard to the woman, her baby, and health care staff.

RUBELLA

The frequency of congenital infection after maternal rubella with a rash is

>80% in the first trimester
50% at 13–14 weeks
25% at the end of the second trimester

Rubella-associated defects are present in almost all infants infected before 11 weeks (mainly cardiac lesions and deafness), and in 35% of those infected at 13–16 weeks (mainly deafness). Infection after 16 weeks is not usually associated with defects.

Among the congenital defects associated (singly or in combination) with maternal rubella are:

Cardiac lesions of many kinds
Eye lesions — cataract, chorio-retinitis, microphthalmia,

glaucoma
Deafness
Expanded syndrome involving the liver, spleen, brain and skeleton which may lead to abortion, stillbirth, IUGR, microcephaly, or mental retardation

Management after maternal exposure

1. Check radial haemolytic (RH) antibodies. High titres within the incubation period (14 to 21 days) suggest protection
2. If there is no antibody or only low titres repeat the tests 25 to 28 days after exposure; a rise in titre of four-fold or more confirms recent infection

Only laboratory tests can confirm that a rash is due to rubella. The value of gamma-globulin in preventing infection is doubtful. CVS (see p. 41) can be used to locate the rubella virus in the placenta/fetus by *in situ* hybridisation.

Rubella vaccination

Antenatal testing for rubella antibody should be routine even when noted to be positive in a previous pregnancy. Non-immune women should be offered vaccination within 7 days of delivery. The vaccine is a live-attenuated virus and must not be used during pregnancy or steroid therapy. A vaccinated woman should avoid pregnancy for 3 months, although no cases of fetal rubella infection have been noted after vaccination.

CYTOMEGALOVIRUS (CMV)

CMV is the commonest primary viral infection of pregnant women. It is usually subclinical (95%). It may account for 10 per cent of mental retardation in children up to 6 years of age. Among other consequences are:

Generalised effects:	abortion, stillbirth, IUGR, failure to thrive
Neurological effects:	microcephaly, cerebral palsy, optic atrophy, deafness
Other effects:	thrombocytopenic purpura, jaundice, pneumonia

However, of congenitally infected infants, less than 10% have serious handicaps, and only a minority of these could be detected before 28 weeks.

Congenital infection follows primary (75%) or reinfection (25%) of the mother. It is therefore unlike rubella where only primary infection causes problems. The virus is excreted in breast milk.

Routine screening of pregnant women to detect evidence of primary infection is not clinically useful.

Only CMV-negative blood should be used for transfusion in sero-negative pregnant women and all newborn infants.

OTHER VIRAL INFECTIONS

Varicella zoster infections are uncommon during child-bearing years but can be severe. The fetus can be affected. Zoster immune globulin should be given to affected women in early pregnancy and to the infants of women affected in late pregnancy.

Infection with *human parvovirus B19* is associated with miscarriage and is a recognised cause of non-immune hydrops fetalis. The fetus is unaffected in over 80% of maternal infections.

BETA-HAEMOLYTIC *STREPTOCOCCUS*

Infants of mothers whose genital tract is colonised antenatally with β-haemolytic streptococci are always themselves colonised, but only 1% will be affected by it. Despite this low figure β-HS infections are a significant cause of death in neonatal intensive-care units.

Culture of vaginal swabs from all pregnant women and treatment of all carriers (and their partners) with penicillin is neither effective, practical nor advisable.

The presence of β-HS in the vagina after premature rupture of the membranes may be an indication for delivery and treatment of the infant.

TOXOPLASMOSIS

Caused by a protozoon, *Toxoplasma gondii*. In the UK the incidence of infection in pregnant women is about 2/1000. The

Time of infection	*Risk of fetal transmission*	*Risk of abortion/fetal death if infected*	*Risk of congenital disease*
During first trimester	About 10 %	Fetal death or severe disease (e.g. hydrocephalus, chorioretinitis, and cerebral calcification) likely	
During second trimester	Frequent	Low	High
During third trimester	Very frequent	None	Low risk at or shortly after birth but 80% develop chorioretinitis in later years; severe symptoms rare

best policy is prevention by avoiding undercooked meat, unpasteurised milk, and contact with cat litter; washing all garden produce well and hands after gardening. The risks vary according to gestational age at infection, as shown in the table on page 104.

Testing the mother
Maternal infection is impossible to diagnose clinically because it is either asymptomatic or confused with pregnancy symptoms or 'flu'. Serological testing should be carried out on suspicion, looking for specific IgM antibody. Send sample to *Toxoplasma* Reference Laboratory (TRL). If positive, repeat for confirmation and rising antibody titres. Routine screening needs to be considered but is not performed in the UK because:

1. The incidence of infection is 'low' (but greater than for congenital syphilis for which screening is carried out)
2. A negative test at booking would need to be repeated later in pregnancy
3. It is said not to be 'cost effective'

If current infection is confirmed:

1. Treat with spiramycin for the remainder of pregnancy. Appropriate treatment will reduce transplacental infection by 60% (but not eradicate it)
2. Treat the fetus for infection

Testing and treating the fetus

1. Carry out amniocentesis and cordocentesis and send amniotic fluid and fetal blood to TRL. Infection is confirmed if above samples contain IgM antibodies or if inoculated mice are found to have *T. gondii* (takes up to six weeks)
2. Check for ventricular dilatation by ultrasound at 20–22 weeks
3. If the fetus is infected and ventricular dilatation is present counsel couple regarding termination
4. If fetus infected but seems normal, or parents do not wish to consider termination, treat with pyrimethamine, sulphadiazine and folinic acid for 3 weeks alternating with spiramycin for three weeks for remainder of pregnancy
5. Continue ultrasound monitoring of ventricles

After birth

1. Send samples of placenta, amniotic fluid, cord and maternal blood for serology
2. Carry out detailed clinical examination including cranial X-ray and ultrasound and ophthalmoscopy
3. If toxoplasmosis suspected treat as above for a year. A further pregnancy can be embarked on once the anti-*Toxoplasma* IgM has disappeared. This can take from 6 months to 2 years

LISTERIOSIS

Caused by *Listeria monocytogenes*, which is widely distributed. Most of us are colonised but only in the susceptible (immunocompromised, newborn, elderly and pregnant women) does it cause disease. *The source* is usually dairy products, vegetables, meat and meat products (e.g. paté), poultry or shellfish. Pasteurisation may not eradicate the organism. It thrives at 4°C. There has been a marked increase in cases in recent years. The rate of listeriosis is about 1 in 10 000 births in the UK. It should be considered in all cases of pyrexia of unknown origin in pregnancy, particularly if the amniotic fluid is meconium stained. If suspected, take vaginal swabs for Gram staining and culture, and blood cultures. After birth, the placenta should be examined for the organism. It can cause miscarriage, intrauterine death or pre-term labour. A live-born infant may develop a generalised infection, including meningitis and pneumonia. The organism is sensitive to a wide range of antibiotics including ampicillin.

MALARIA

Malaria must be considered in non-endemic areas among immigrants or tourists returning from endemic areas suffering from unexplained pyrexia. Parasites are seen on thick and thin blood smears. For treatment use chloroquine.

SUGGESTED FURTHER READING

Marwood I 1990 HIV infection and pregnancy. British Journal of Hospital Medicine 43: 287–289

Turnbull A, Chamberlain G (eds) 1989 Obstetrics. Churchill Livingstone, Edinburgh

Problems in later pregnancy

ANTEPARTUM HAEMORRHAGE

Definition

Bleeding from the genital tract from 28 completed weeks of pregnancy to the birth of the baby, including the first and second stages of labour.

Sources

1. Separation of a placenta lying partly or wholly within the lower uterine segment — *placenta praevia*
2. Separation of a normally situated placenta — *abruptio placentae*
3. Lesions of the cervix or vagina
4. Unknown

Incidence

Approximately 3% of pregnancies progressing beyond 28 weeks' gestation.

PLACENTA PRAEVIA

Clinical features

Vaginal bleeding — slight, moderate or heavy, most commonly occurring between 32 and 37 weeks' gestation. It may have been preceded by several slight 'warning haemorrhages'. The bleeding is usually painless (in the absence of labour). The abdomen is usually soft and non-tender to palpation. Fetal parts are readily palpable, and the fetal heart can be heard. If the placenta is praevia and anterior, the presenting part may be difficult to palpate. The presenting part is high, or the lie is oblique or transverse; breech presentation is common. (A persistently high presenting part or variable lie should raise the suspicion of *placenta praevia* even in the absence of vaginal bleeding.)

Management

1. From home: organise immediate admission. *Do not perform a vaginal examination* because it may provoke profuse bleeding. Stop oral intake — she may need an anaesthetic
2. In hospital: manage expectantly if haemorrhage is not severe and pregnancy has not reached 36 to 37 weeks
   - (i) Localise placenta by ultrasound (see below)
   - (ii) A gentle speculum examination can be carried out when bleeding has ceased for at least 24 hours
   - (iii) Keep two units of blood cross-matched as clinical judgement dictates
   - (iv) If bleeding continues make sure that the blood is maternal rather than fetal using Apt's test which distinguishes between them on the basis that fetal haemoglobin is relatively resistant to denaturation
   - (v) Check for feto-maternal transfusion in Rh-D-negative women and give anti-D immunoglobulin as necessary
   - (vi) Monitor fetal welfare (see p. 45)
   - (vii) If the diagnosis of significant placenta praevia is confirmed the patient should remain in hospital

Indications for intervention

1. Heavy bleeding or continuous oozing is compromising maternal or fetal health
2. Moderate or heavy bleeding occurs when the pregnancy has reached 37 completed weeks or more
3. Expectant management has allowed the pregnancy to reach 38 weeks

Mode of intervention

If the diagnosis of a major degree of placenta praevia is certain and maternal and/or fetal health are in jeopardy, or if there is a malpresentation carry out Caesarean section.

If there is some doubt as to the diagnosis, the degree of placenta praevia is minor, and the fetus presents by the vertex, carry out an examination in the theatre set for Caesarean section.

If placenta praevia is confirmed proceed to Caesarean section; if not, an amniotomy can be performed. If the cervix is unfavourable and the fetus is in good condition it may be justifiable to allow the pregnancy to proceed to term.

Note: There is an increased risk of postpartum haemorrhage when the placenta has encroached on the lower segment.

Localisation of the placenta

Ultrasound is the method of choice.

If a low-lying placenta is detected early in pregnancy the scans should be repeated later in pregnancy because the placenta may seem to 'migrate' away from the lower segment as it forms in late pregnancy. Only 1 in 10 placentae thought to be low-lying early in pregnancy persists as clinically relevant placenta praevia towards term.

A low-lying placenta discovered during an ultrasound examination for another reason and in the absence of bleeding can be managed as follows:

(i) Before 28 weeks — repeat the scan in 1 month
(ii) After 28 weeks — discuss the findings with the patient and advise her to avoid coitus. If she lives a long distance from the hospital, or if there are other adverse circumstances, it may be advisable to admit her to hospital. Repeat the scan each month

ABRUPTIO PLACENTAE

The haemorrhage arises from one or more maternal spiral arterioles retroplacentally. Its incidence has fallen over recent years.

Revealed haemorrhage — the blood tracks between the membrane and the uterine wall and escapes at the introitus.

Concealed haemorrhage — a large haematoma forms between the placenta and the uterus. No external bleeding occurs.

Mixed haemorrhage — combines features of the above. It is the commonest.

Associated factors

1. High parity and poor nutrition
2. Hypertension and pre-eclampsia
3. Sudden reduction in uterine volume, e.g. when a patient with hydramnios loses a large volume of liquor
4. External cephalic version (occasionally) particularly if carried out under general anaesthesia
5. Trauma (rarely)
6. Previous abruption
7. Unknown

Clinical features of severe placental abruption

Intense, constant abdominal pain with or without vaginal bleeding
A degree of shock out of proportion to extent of blood loss
Tender uterus perhaps large for dates and increasing in size
Fetal parts may be difficult to feel
Fetal heart sounds may be irregular or absent
Proteinuria
Coagulation defect may develop
Oliguria or anuria in really severe cases

Differential diagnosis

1. Placenta praevia
2. Uterine rupture
3. Degeneration of a fibroid
4. Rectus sheath haematoma
5. Acute hydramnios
6. Acute surgical conditions

Management

1. Single episode of slight bleeding, mother and fetus in good condition and before 36 weeks' gestation. Manage conservatively (as for placenta praevia) and monitor fetal welfare regularly (see p. 45). Induce labour if indicated at 38 to 40 weeks.
2. Severe abruption
   (i) Begin resuscitation at home before transfer to hospital
   (ii) Admit by ambulance accompanied by GP or midwife or by Flying Squad
   (iii) Correct shock and hypovolaemia with intravenous fluids. Monitor central venous pressure and urine volume
   (iv) Expedite delivery by amniotomy and judicious oxytocin
   (v) Monitor FHR continuously — an acidotic (hypoxic) fetus should be delivered by Caesarean section
   (vi) A case can be made for Caesarean section in some cases in which the fetus is already dead such as when the cervix is tightly shut and amniotomy is impossible; e.g. there is, as yet, no coagulation defect but if the uterus were not to be emptied quickly the risk of it developing would be high
   (vii) Check for coagulation defect and platelet count
   (viii) Beware of postpartum haemorrhage. Hysterectomy may be necessary in some rare circumstances. It must neither be carried out too soon nor too late! The judgement of a senior obstetrician is mandatory

Complications of abruptio placentae

1. Coagulation failure (see p. 149)
2. Post-partum haemorrhage (see p. 145)
3. Renal failure. Acute tubular necrosis may result from hypovolaemia and intravascular coagulation within the kidney.
   (i) Control fluid and electrolyte balance
   (ii) Tubular necrosis is best prevented by early and adequate correction of shock with intravenous fluids and blood
   (iii) Forced diuresis is not indicated

(iv) Renal dialysis may be necessary temporarily
Recovery of renal function is to be expected

OTHER CAUSES OF ANTEPARTUM HAEMORRHAGE

Local causes, e.g.:
1. Vaginitis
2. Cervical polyp
3. Cervical ectropion
4. Carcinoma of cervix

A gentle speculum examination will help to detect these.

Unknown cause
Do not ignore antepartum haemorrhage even if its cause cannot be determined. There is a high incidence of pre-term delivery in this group. Fetal welfare should be monitored for the remainder of pregnancy with the patient in or out of hospital as clinical circumstances dictate.

POLYHYDRAMNIOS

Definition
An excessive volume of amniotic. It can be chronic or acute: the latter can mimic abruptio placentae.

Associated features
1. Maternal diabetes
2. Multiple pregnancy (especially monovular twins)
3. Fetal anomaly, e.g. neural tube defect, oesophageal atresia,
4. Hydrops fetalis

Consequences
1. Maternal discomfort
2. Unstable lie of the fetus
3. Increased incidence of pre-term labour
4. If the membranes rupture prematurely the following may happen:
   (i) Prolapsed cord
   (ii) Malpresentation of fetus
   (iii) Placental abruption

Management
Check random blood sugar in all except minor cases.

Carry out ultrasound scan and/or abdominal X-ray to exclude those fetal anomalies amenable to diagnosis

Tapping of fluid in severe cases produces only brief respite and may induce pre-term labour.

In diabetic women tighter control of the diabetes may cause some lessening of fluid volume.

Diuretics are of no value.

Test the infant for oesophageal atresia at birth.

HYDROPS FETALIS

Definition

The accumulation of fluid in some or all of the serous cavities in the fetus accompanied by generalised oedema of the skin. The placenta may also be oedematous. Fetal ascites can be an early manifestation.

Clinical aspects

The commonest presenting features are polyhydramnios or a large-for-dates uterus. However, the uterus may be small-for-dates and oligohydramnios be present.

There may be associated pre-eclampsia or severe anaemia.

Causes

Among the best recognised causes are:

1. Rhesus iso-immunisation — at one time the commonest, now rare (see p. 88)
2. Cardiovascular lesions — e.g. many cardiac anomalies, congenital heart block, tachydysrhythmias
3. Chromosomal disorders — e.g. trisomies (particularly trisomy 21), Turner syndrome, triploidy
4. Congenital malformations — e.g. several recognised syndromes, diaphragmatic herniae, bladder neck obstruction
5. Haematological — e.g. beta-thalassaemia, glucose-6-phosphate dehydrogenase deficiency
6. Twin–twin transfusion syndrome
7. Infections e.g. parvovirus, CMV, toxoplasmosis, rubella, syphilis
8. Placental and umbilical cord lesions — chorioangioma, feto-maternal transfusion, umbilical vein thrombosis
9. Maternal conditions — severe diabetes or anaemia, hypoproteinaemia

In 15–30% of cases a cause is not identifiable.

Investigation

Antenatal detection is possible in most cases.

1. Ultrasound is the most important for initial detection and subsequent assessment
2. Maternal blood — blood group and antibodies; and to exclude G-6-PD deficiency, beta-thalassaemia, infection and Kleihauer test
3. Fetal heart monitoring and echocardiography may be helpful

4. Amniocentesis — karyotype; amniotic fluid AFP, CMV culture, and specific metabolic tests
5. Cordocentesis (see p. 41) — fetal blood for IgM, karyotype, DNA analysis and metabolic tests

Management
This depends on the cause and severity of the condition. In general the prognosis is poor, particularly if fetal movements are reduced. For fetal therapy see p. 43.

MALPRESENTATIONS

1. High head at term
Though not strictly a malpresentation it may develop into one during labour. It is common in multiparous patients, but potential causes must be considered in primigravidae.

Causes
(i) Greater than average angle of inclination of the brim, e.g. in Negro patients
(ii) A deflexed head
(iii) Head too large to enter pelvis easily — hydrocephalus: large baby
(iv) Pelvis too small
(v) There is something in the way — placenta praevia, fibroid, the head of an undiagnosed twin
(vi) Too much room for movement, e.g. hydramnios
(vii) No abnormality whatsoever — in one-third of all primigravidae the head remains unengaged (though perhaps not 'high') at term

Management
If a significant cause can be ruled out there is no cause for concern.

2. Variable lie towards term
If the fetal lie is persistently variable after 37 weeks' gestation the woman should be admitted.

Exclude causes such as wrong dates, placenta praevia, multiple pregnancy, and pelvic tumour.

If the lie stabilises to longitudinal she can be allowed home or labour can be induced at term.

If the variable lie persists to 41 weeks carry out an elective Caesarean section.

3. Breech presentation (see p. 133)

4. Face and brow presentation (see p. 137)

MULTIPLE PREGNANCY

The incidence of twin pregnancy has fallen from about 1:80 to 1:100 pregnancies, but there are marked geographical and regional variations.

The incidence of triplets is still about $1:80^2$ and of quadruplets about $1:80^3$.

Twinning

Monovular — identical
Binovular — fraternal (familial tendency)

Types of monovular twins

1. *Dichorial, diamniotic* — about 30% of twins; the zygote separates at the two-cell stage
2. *Monochorial, diamniotic* — about 70% of twins. Twinning occurs within the blastocyst and the placentae anastomose to a variable extent. One twin may monopolise the placental circulation
3. *Monochorial, monoamniotic* — about 1% of twins. A single amniotic sac invests both and the yolk sac is divided into two. The placental circulations anastomose completely and the umbilical cords may become intertwined
4. *Conjoint twins* — 1% of monozygotic twins; all are monochorial, monoamniotic. The extent of the conjunction is variable

Histological confirmation of monovularity or binovularity is necessary after delivery.

Clinical features

Ten per cent of multiple pregnancies are missed by early scans, and an early scan showing two (or more) gestation sacs may not progress as a multiple pregnancy.

All the hazards of pregnancy are increased, particularly anaemia, pre-eclampsia, hydramnios, pre-term labour and intrapartum problems.

Iron and folic acid supplements are necessary.

Ten per cent of all pre-term labours are associated with multiple pregnancy.

Routine admission at 26 to 30 or 30 to 34 weeks is not indicated. Admit if:

1. Any complications supervene (e.g. pre-eclampsia)
2. The cervix is effacing too soon
3. The mother is excessively tired

Prophylactic oral beta-sympathomimetic drugs do not reduce the risk of pre-term labour.

Check fetal growth and welfare antenatally by serial ultrasound and BPP scoring.

If the pregnancy reaches 40 weeks' gestation labour can be induced to reduce the risk from any placental insufficiency.

POST-TERM PREGNANCY

A pregnancy is post-term when it extends beyond 293 days (42 weeks) from the first day of the LMP. The extent of fetal risk from this degree of post-maturity is controversial. At most, 0.5% of all perinatal deaths are attributed to it. The risk is counterbalanced by risks of induction and of possible errors in dates leading to the delivery of a pre-term infant. Ultrasound dating in early pregnancy reduces the latter risk.

Induction of labour should not be a matter of mere routine in the absence of other complications. The mother's opinion should be considered and the state of the cervix taken into account.

THE MANAGEMENT OF INTRAUTERINE FETAL DEATH (IUFD)

Causes (see p. 152)

Diagnosis

Ultrasound — no fetal heart or movement can be detected and there is overlap of skull bones in the absence of labour.

Management

Induction of labour by amniotomy is absolutely contra-indicated in the presence of an IUFD because of the risk of overwhelming intrauterine infection.

Oxytocin infusions alone are ineffective.

Intravenous prostaglandins have severe side-effects (vomiting and diarrhoea).

Extra-amniotic prostaglandins require expertise.

The alternative is vaginal prostaglandin E_2 (up to 28 weeks uterine size 15 mg; after 28 weeks uterine size 5 mg).

If delivery is not complete within 12 hours set up an oxytocin infusion.

Sensitive and sympathetic support for the mother and family are vital (see p. 154).

SUGGESTED FURTHER READING

Baskett T F 1985 Essential management of obstetric emergencies. John Wiley, Chichester

MacGillivray I, Campbell D M, Thompson B (eds) 1988 Twinning and twins. Wiley, Chichester

Turnbull A, Chamberlain G (eds) 1989 Obstetrics. Churchill Livingstone, Edinburgh

Labour and intrapartum problems

PHYSIOLOGY OF PARTURITION

1. *Uterine growth* is stimulated by mechanical stretching and oestrogens. New muscle forms only in early pregnancy; hypertrophy occurs in mid-pregnancy and distension thereafter
2. *Uterine activity before labour*. Uterine muscle contracts rhythmically even when isolated. As they contract, myometrial fibres also retract (i.e. they preserve the same tone but shorten). This is the mechanism by which the physiological lower segment forms late in pregnancy and cervical dilatation occurs during labour.

   Progesterone blocks myometrial excitability; sensitivity to oxytocin increases as pregnancy advances; responses to PGs are the same throughout.

   Uterine contractions during the first 20 weeks are of high frequency but low intensity. Frequency and amplitude increase thereafter. Irregular, low-frequency, high-amplitude (Braxton–Hicks) contractions are most apparent in the last two months.

   As labour approaches the activity of the fundal myometrium increases most while the lower segment remains relatively inactive. The cervix thus becomes effaced, and engagement of the presenting part is encouraged.

INITIATION OF LABOUR

Maternal and feto-placental factors may be involved in the onset of spontaneous labour.

Maternal factors

1. *Myometrium*

   This remains relatively quiescent despite massive stretching due to the action of progesterone. Removal of this block (see below) may facilitate the onset of labour. The role of α (stimulatory) and β (inhibitory) adrenergic receptors in initiating labour are uncertain. PGs are involved locally in

the action of the myometrial cell but are probably not the primary stimulus
2. *Decidua* is a prime source of prostaglandins
3. The *posterior pituitary gland* produces oxytocin but there is no increase in levels before the onset of labour

Feto-placental factors

1. *The placenta*
   In many animals progesterone levels fall as oestrogens rise near the onset of labour. Oestrogen stimulates PG production (see below) and the fall in progesterone increases myometrial excitability. Unfortunately the change in the oestrogen/progesterone ratio is much less in humans and no direct relationship between changes and the onset of labour has been shown
2. *Fetal membranes*
   The amnion is a potent source of PGs
3. *Fetal pituitary adrenal axis*
   Throughout most of fetal life the main products of the fetal anterior pituitary are the peptide fragments of ACTH known as α-MSH (α-melanotrophin) and CLIP (corticotrophin-like intermediate lobe peptide) which drive the fetal zone of the adrenal. A switch occurs to intact ACTH near term which stimulates development of the definitive adrenal cortex. The production of cortisol by ACTH is important in the initiation of labour in several species (e.g. sheep) but is not essential in man. Prolactin is the second trophic agent for the fetal adrenal and it encourages oestrogen production

Possible sequence of events

1. Progesterone-binding protein increases at term: the tissue effects of progesterone decrease
2. The suppression of myometrial excitability by progesterone decreases
3. The relative fall in progesterone also promotes the release of arachidonic acid
4. ACTH promotes DHEA production in the fetal adrenal which goes on to form oestrone and oestradiol
5. Oestrogens further stimulate the production of arachidonic acid
6. PGs are produced in decidua and fetal membranes
7. Labour is initiated

NORMAL LABOUR

Normal labour is characterised by
(i) Regular uterine contractions
(ii) Dilatation of the cervix
(iii) Descent of the presenting part

It encompasses the time from the onset of regular contractions to spontaneous vaginal delivery of the infant (within 24 hours).

Uterine contractions
Contractions begin in two 'pace-makers' near the uterotubal junctions. Only one is operative in each contraction which spreads like a wave over the whole uterus. Relaxation begins simultaneously in all areas of the uterus. Labour is characterised by:

Strong and sustained action of the muscle of the uterine fundus
Less strong contractions of the mid-zone
Relative inactivity of the lower segment

This fundal dominance increases as labour progresses.

Cervical dilatation
This occurs from above downwards accompanied by effacement (thinning).

It is caused by co-ordinated contraction and retraction of the upper segment. The forewaters may act as a hydrostatic wedge, and dilatation is facilitated by close apposition of the cervix and presenting part.

First stage of labour
Latent and active phases
The latent phase starts from the onset of regular uterine contractions and ends when the cervix is 2 to 3 cm dilated and fully effaced. It occurs because the thinning of the lower

CERVICAL DILATATION TIME CURVE

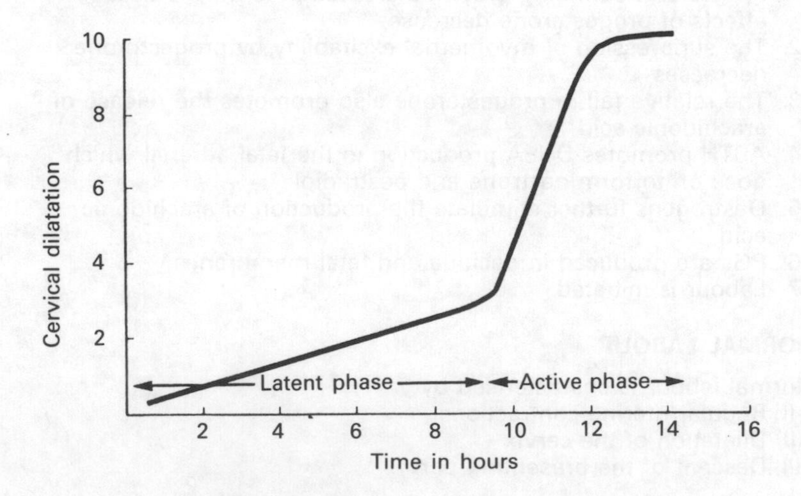

segment and cervix take a lot of uterine work before rapid dilatation can begin.
In the active phase the cervix dilates at 1 to 3 cm per hour in primigravidae and up to 6 cm per hour in multigravidae.

Length of first stage of labour

	Mean length in hours (± 1 SD)	
	Primigravidae	*Multigravidae*
Latent phase	9 ± 6	5 ± 4
Active phase	5 ± 3.5	2 ±1.5

Control of uterine activity in labour
Prostaglandins are, and oxytocin may be, important for the maintenance of progressive labour.

The autonomic nervous system has little or no motor function.

Progress in labour is best assessed using a partogram on which can be recorded:

1. Cervical dilatation — marked in centimetres at zero time (the time of admission to labour ward) and at every subsequent examination
2. Descent of the head (in fifths palpable above the pelvic brim)
3. Contractions — frequency, duration and strength assessed for 10 minutes each ½ hour. Normal uterine contractions are characterised by:
   (i) A frequency of one every 2 to 3 minutes with at least 1 minute between contractions
   (ii) A duration of 40 to 70 seconds
   (iii) An intensity (measured by intrauterine catheter) of around 50 mmHg with a resting tonus of <10 mmHg
4. Fetal heart rate (see p. 130)
5. Condition of the liquor and time and manner of membrane rupture
6. Moulding of the fetal skull
7. Dosage of oxytocin, if used
8. Maternal status (BP, pulse, temperature, urinalysis) and medication

Management of normal labour
Each obstetric unit must set down agreed guidelines for the management of labour. These must begin with a clear statement about the diagnosis of the onset of labour.

Posture
Mobility should be encouraged during the latent phase. In the active phase (in the absence of complications) allow the mother to adopt the position she finds most comfortable. Maternal posture should at all times be as upright as possible to enhance placental perfusion

Normal progress
In primigravidae delivery should be expected within 8 hours of the diagnosis of labour and achieved within 12 hours. Delay in primigravid labour may be due to:
(i) Inefficient uterine action
(ii) Occipito-posterior position of the fetal head
(iii) True cephalo-pelvic disproportion (rarely)
Labour is much more rapid in multiparous women, and inefficient uterine action is rare. If delay is occuring its cause should be sought and corrected if possible. Prolonged labour in a multiparous woman is likely to be due to obstruction.

Augmentation of labour in primigravidae

Indications
If the rate of cervical dilatation is less than 1 cm per hour in the active phase of labour.

Technique
The membranes are ruptured and oxytocin infusion is set up 1 hour later if labour does not accelerate.

Aim
To achieve safe delivery within 8 hours of admission to the labour ward.

Contra-indications
1. In the presence of obstetric anomalies, e.g. breech presentation or multiple pregnancy.
2. In the face of fetal compromise.

Augmentation of labour in multigravidae must not be routine because the risk of uterine rupture is high.

Oral intake in labour
Food and drink can be given to a mother during labour provided that:
1. She has received no narcotic analgesia (or at most one small dose of pethidine)
2. She is not becoming excessively tired (these two factors increase gastric stasis)
3. Only low-fat, low-residue food is given

Ketonuria is present in up to 40% of normal labours when tested by Ketostix. Its significance is exaggerated and it is over-treated in labouring women. Few women with ketonuria are dehydrated, acidaemic or hypoglycaemic. Clinically significant ketosis is very unlikely to occur in the first 12 hours of labour and intravenous therapy is usually within that time.

Intravenous infusions of dextrose solutions (particularly dextrose 10% are contra-indicated because of their deleterious effect on mother and baby.
If dehydration needs to be corrected, normal saline should be infused and the volume must not exceed 3 litres/24 hours.

Second stage of labour

1. It begins with full dilatation of the cervix and ends with delivery of the baby
2. Its average length in primigravidae is 40 minutes, and in multiparae is 20 minutes
3. It has two phases — the *propulsive phase* from full dilatation until the presenting part has descended to the pelvic floor, and the *expulsive phase* which ends with delivery of the baby and is recognised by the mother's irresistible desire to bear down and/or distension of the perineum

A woman should not usually be encouraged to bear down until she has entered the expulsive phase. A prolonged propulsive phase in primigravidae due to inefficient uterine action (and not cephalo-pelvic disproportion) can be treated judiciously with oxytocin.

INDUCTION OF LABOUR

Indications

1. When the intrauterine risks to the fetus are such that he or she will be safer delivered
2. When the risk to the mother's health from the continuation of pregnancy outweighs the risk to the fetus from delivery

If the added risk of labour is unacceptable, delivery must be by Caesarean section.

Otherwise, labour can be induced and the maternal and fetal state monitored throughout.

The optimum time for delivery is often difficult to judge, and secure knowledge of gestational age is important.

Social indications rarely constitute an adequate reason for induction but each situation must be considered on its merits.

Contra-indications

1. Absolute

1. The fetal lie is not longitudinal
2. Caesarean section has been carried out in a previous pregnancy for a recurrent reason, e.g. pelvic contraction
3. Two previous Caesarean sections have been performed
4. A tumour occupies the pelvis

2. Relative
1. The cervix has previously been repaired. Previous cone biopsy merits caution
2. Highly multiparous woman

3. Other factors to be borne in mind
1. An unfavourable cervix
2. Uncertain gestational age

Hazards
1. Iatrogenic prematurity — early pregnancy dating by ultrasound reduces this risk
2. Infection — there is little appreciable risk in practice but amnionitis can always be detected within 36 hours of amniotomy.
3. Neonatal jaundice — there is a small risk if the total dose of oxytocin exceeds 20 units
4. Failed induction — defined as failure to deliver vaginally a patient in whom safe vaginal delivery was expected. The incidence is not less than 2% of all inductions
5. Additional hazards — induced labours are longer, require more analgesia, have a higher incidence of instrumental delivery and Caesarean section, and lower Apgar scores than comparable spontaneous labours

Cervical ripeness
This is assessed by a 'Bishop score' which gives marks of 0 to 3 for five cervical features:
1. Dilatation (cm)
2. Length (cm)
3. Station of head (cm above ischial spines)
4. Consistency
5. Position

If the cervix is 'ripe' (score >5) induction of labour is likely to be successful. With a score of <5 induction is more likely to fail, the latent phase will tend to be longer, and a higher total dose of oxytocin will be necessary to reach optimal uterine activity.

The cervix can be ripened with prostaglandin E_2 (inserted into the vagina on the morning of induction (dose: multipara 2.5 to 3 mg, primigravida 5 to 6 mg). Hyperstimulation of the uterus is rare but can occur. Frequent low-amplitude contractions within 20 minutes of insertion are common.

Fetal heart rate monitoring is advisable if induction is being carried out for fetal reasons.

Methods of induction
1. Vaginal prostaglandin — the above regime may induce labour, particularly in women with a favourable cervix

2. Amniotomy
3. Oxytocin infusion by peristaltic or syringe pump

The dose of oxytocin required to produce effective uterine action is between 4 and 16 milliunits per minute (mu/min). Occasionally as much as 32 mu/min are necessary. As labour becomes established the uterus becomes more sensitive to oxytocin and the effective dose rate reduces to about 8 mu/min.

Actual regimes are numerous but each must follow the following principles:

1. Low doses initially, gradually increasing to produce effective contractions
2. Dose rate varied to suit the individual woman
3. Any complications such as hyperstimulation must be detected early

Water intoxication has occasionally followed the infusion of large volumes of oxytocin containing fluid. Confusion and convulsions can proceed to coma and even death. This is totally avoidable.

PAIN IN LABOUR

Pain is a normal part of labour and delivery although emotional, cultural and other influences alter individual responses.

1. Causes
   (i) Dilatation of the cervix
   (ii) Contraction and distension of the uterus, possibly due to the accumulation of pain-producing substances during ischaemia
   (iii) Distension of vagina and perineum
   (iv) Pressure on other organs (e.g. bladder and rectum) or the lumbosacral plexus; spasm in skeletal muscles
2. Sensory pathways are T10 to L1 for both uterine body and cervix

	T10	
Stimulated during latent phase when pain not severe }	T11	stimulated during
	T12	active phase
	L1	

   Referred pain is experienced in the dermatomes of the above segments.
3. Factors affecting pain in childbirth
   Physical factors including:
   (i) Intensity and duration of contractions
   (ii) Speed of dilatation of cervix
   (iii) Vaginal and perineal distension
   (iv) Other factors e.g. age, parity, size of infant, condition of patient
   Physiological factors:
   (i) Pain blocking e.g. customs, culture, preparation, distractive activity

(ii) Pain aggravating e.g. customs, culture, fear, apprehension, anxiety, ignorance, misinformation
(iii) Antenatal preparation of the mother and father are very important

(The common midwifery practice of massaging the skin of the lower back or abdomen modulates pain perception.)

ANALGESIA

Antenatal education is a vital part of preparing women for the pain of labour.

Methods for pain relief

1. *Psychological methods* to counteract the 'fear–tension' sequence. Pain-relieving drugs can be used to supplement the mother's own efforts.
   With proper training, 30 to 40% of women can go through labour without requiring analgesic drugs
2. *Narcotic drugs*, e.g. pethidine, by intramuscular injection. The first injection is often combined with a phenothiazine, e.g. promazine or promethazine to add to the analgesic effect and decrease nausea and vomiting. They may produce maternal and fetal tachycardia.
   Advantages
   (i) Ease of administration
   (ii) Reasonably rapid analgesia
   (iii) Low incidence of serious side-effects
   (iv) Antagonists available
   Disadvantages
   (i) Inadequate analgesia in up to 40% of patients
   (ii) Nausea and vomiting common
   (iii) Psychic disturbances common, e.g. confusion, inability to cooperate
   (iv) Delayed gastric emptying
   (v) Neonatal respiratory depression
   Contra-indications
   (i) Previous idiosyncratic reactions
   (ii) Current mono-amine oxidase inhibitors
3. Inhalational agents
   Nitrous oxide (50%) and oxygen (50%) — 'Entonox' apparatus
   Inhalational agents are usually used too late and too hesitantly. They can be highly effective and safe for mother and baby
4. *Epidural analgesia*. Lumbar or caudal analgesia will provide total or adequate analgesia in up to 90% of patients.
   Indications. If epidural analgesia is not available on request it may be helpful for:

(i) Prolonged labour
(ii) Breech presentation
(iii) Multiple pregnancy
(iv) Pre-term labour
(v) Forceps delivery (particulary rotational)
(vi) Hypertension in labour — close supervision is vital
(vii) Vaginismus

Contraindications

(i) Lack of experienced personnel
(ii) Infection at the injection site
(iii) Bony abnormalities of the spinal column
(iv) Coagulation defects or bleeding diathesis
(v) Anticoagulant therapy
(vi) Hypovolaemia
(vii) Active neurological disease
(viii) Idiosyncratic reactions to local anaesthetic agents

Immediate maternal hazards

(i) Dural tap — dural puncture by needle or catheter; it leads to 'spinal' headache (see below)
(ii) Total spinal — loss of all sensory and motor function; can include unconsciousness, severe hypotension and apnoea; it results from subarachnoid injection of epidural dose of local anaesthetic agent
(iii) Hypotension — can be avoided by nursing the patient on her side and by the intravenous infusion of Hartmann's solution before the block is established (also used for treatment of hypotension)
(iv) Motor paralysis — reduces maternal expulsive effort, tends to prevent rotation of the fetal head and makes instrumental delivery more likely
(v) Toxic reactions to local anaesthetic agents

Delayed maternal hazards

(i) Severe spinal headache due to spinal tap. Management: (a) keep patient lying down; (b) slow intra-injection of 1.0 to 1.5 l normal saline for 24 h;
(ii) 'Blood patch' — injection of 10 ml autologous blood into epidural space
(ii) Urinary retention — more usually due to method and circumstances of delivery
(iii) Sepsis — extremely unlikely if bacterial filter is used
(iv) Temporary diminished sensation of dermatomes affected

Backache may be caused by epidural analgesia.

Fetal effects

There are no direct adverse effects on the fetus.

Guidelines

The regional block may be continuous during labour or as a single injection for operative delivery.

Bupivacaine (0.5, 0.375 or 0.25%) is the preferred anaesthetic — a test dose should be injected initially.

Constant monitoring of maternal and fetal condition is mandatory.

Top-up dose must be individually chosen when the patient begins to experience discomfort

Epidural analgesia and previous Caesarean section

Epidural block is permissible in any woman who is being allowed to labour having previously been delivered by Caesarean section. FHR and ideally intrauterine pressure should be monitored throughout

5. *Transcutaneous electrical nerve stimulation (TENS).* This aims to reduce pain by stimulating large myelinated nerve fibres to reduce input from small myelinated and non-myelinated fibres linked to peripheral pain receptors. Low-intensity continuous stimulation is applied to the dermatomes associated with the pain. It can provide good to moderate pain relief but success depends on time spent teaching and supporting the mother before and during use.

PRE-TERM LABOUR AND DELIVERY

Definition

Regular, painful uterine contractions accompanied by effacement and dilatation of the cervix after 20 and before 37 completed weeks of pregnancy.

It accounts for 5 to 10% of all deliveries but 85% of neonatal deaths.

Factors associated with pre-term delivery

Spontaneous labour — cause unknown	40%
Spontaneous labour due to maternal or fetal conditions other than multiple pregnancy	25%
Multiple pregnancy	10%
Elective delivery	25%

Causes of spontaneous pre-term labour (roughly in order of importance)

1. Multiple pregnancy
2. Antepartum haemorrhage
3. Intrauterine growth retardation
4. Cervical incompetence
5. Amnionitis
6. Congenital uterine anomaly
7. Diabetes
8. Polyhydramnios
9. Pyelonephritis
10. Other infections

Prediction of risk
No scoring system yet devised has proven itself superior to clinical judgement. The strongest association is with previous pre-term delivery.

Management varies according to five main factors
1. *The state of the membranes.* The efficacy or even advisability of attempts to inhibit pre-term labour when the membranes are ruptured is open to question
2. *Dilatation of the cervix.* Labour is likely to progress if the cervix is >4 cm dilated
3. *Gestational age.* The earlier the gestation, the more strenuous attempts to inhibit labour must be. Labour should be allowed to progress if the estimated fetal weight is >2000 g
4. *The cause of pre-term labour.* If the cause is (or will soon be) prejudicing fetal welfare, delivery is indicated
5. *The availability of neonatal intensive care facilities.* If facilities are inadequate consider transfer of the patient to a unit with better facilities, but do not leave transfer too late

Inhibition of pre-term labour.
In up to 50% of patients contractions will stop spontaneously and the pregnancy will continue to term without any treatment whatsoever. The clinical problem is to discern correctly those in whom drug therapy is indicated. One possible guide is the presence or absence of 'fetal breathing' movements assessed by real-time ultrasound over a maximum of 45 minutes. If fetal breathing is observed the contractions are more likely to subside spontaneously.

1. Beta-sympatomimetic drugs
These drugs, e.g. salbutamol or ritodrine hydrochloride, suppress uterine activity. Prolongation of pregnancy is, however, not necessarily beneficial to the fetus. Each case must be considered on its merits.
Potential side-effects:
Maternal tachycardia
Hypotension
Fetal tachycardia
Palpitations, headache, visual disturbances, skin flushing, nausea and vomiting
Hyperkalaemia
Hyperglycaemia
Rarely right heart failure may develop (usually when glucocorticoids have also been given).
Contra-indications:
Antepartum haemorrhage

Severe pre-eclampsia
Maternal anti-hypertensive therapy (risk of myocardial infarction)
Maternal cardiac disease or thyrotoxicosis
Any other situation in which the prolongation of pregnancy could be hazardous
Extreme caution must be exercised if the woman has diabetes, or is being treated with corticosteroids or potassium-depleting diuretics.

Prophylactic oral betamimetics do not prevent pre-term labour.

2. Calcium channel blockade, e.g. nifedipine (see p. 67)
They do not further reduce BP in normotensive women.

Glucocorticoid therapy and the prevention of hyaline membrane disease
Corticosteroids given to the mother before 34 weeks can induce pulmonary surfactant in the lungs of the immature fetus. One regimen is dexamethasone 12 mg i.m. on two successive days repeated weekly to 32–34 weeks.

Method of delivery in pre-term labour
If the fetus is viable it must be delivered by the route least likely to cause trauma or hypoxia. This may mean Caesarean section but not necessarily so. Caesarean sections at early gestation, and with infants under 1000 g, can be hazardous for the mother, and are not necessarily safer for the baby. The indications for Caesarean section are stronger but not absolute in multiple pregnancy and breech presentation.

Pre-term labour is unpredictable and the woman may become fully-dilated quickly and silently.

PREMATURE RUPTURE OF THE MEMBRANES (PROM)

This is defined as rupture of the membranes before the onset of labour without reference to gestational age. It can be managed conservatively before 34 to 36 week's gestation unless intrauterine infection is present or likely to develop.

A high vaginal swab should be taken on admission. If it grows any significant organisms (particularly beta-haemolytic streptococci), delivery should be expedited and the neonatal paediatricians alerted. Any intrauterine infection must be treated vigorously and expeditiously.

In term pregnancies 90% of women with PROM go into labour within 24 hours and deliver satisfactorily. In the absence of any evidence of infection or cord entanglement the onset of labour can be awaited for 24 (and possibly 48) hours. Labour can be induced in those women who remain undelivered.

INTRAPARTUM FETAL MONITORING

The aim is to detect fetal hypoxia.

Effects of hypoxia depend on the fetal glycogen reserves. A growth-retarded fetus will therefore be affected earlier and more severely than a well-nourished fetus.

1. Anaerobic glycolysis results in an accumulation of lactate. This causes a fetal metabolic acidosis
2. The fetal pCO_2 rises, causing a respiratory acidosis
3. The blood pH falls
4. Fetal heart rate patterns change (see below) the most serious being decelerations

The traditional diagnosis of 'fetal distress' depended predominantly on the crude observation of heart changes. 'Fetal distress' is an imprecise and rather unhelpful term. Half of all babies delivered by forceps or Caesarean section because of 'fetal distress' are not hypoxic; and half of the most hypoxic babies do not exhibit classical signs of 'fetal distress'.

Methods of intrapartum monitoring

1. *Intermittent recording of FHR* using a fetal stethoscope:
   - (i) Between contractions to obtain a baseline rate
   - (ii) During and immediately after contractions to detect accelerations or decelerations. It is applicable only to low-risk patients with no obstetric abnormalities. More intensive monitoring (see below) should be used if any risk factors are present (see below).

2. *Continuous recording of FHR.*

This is best obtained by an electrode attached to fetal scalp (or buttock). The monitor measures the interval between paired beats, converts it into 'beats per minute' (b.p.m) and registers it.

Uterine activity can be assessed by an external strain gauge transducer or measured by intrauterine catheter.

The combined print-out of continuous FHR and uterine activity is a cardiotocograph (CTG). Continuous recording of the FHR is a screening technique which facilitates the detection of fetal hypoxic stress. It is not diagnostic. Even when the most ominous pattern is present (see below) only 50% of the babies have a low Apgar score (see p. 159) at birth. Continuous FHR recordings must therefore be backed up by measurement of fetal scalp pH (see below).

Guide to indications for continuous FHR monitoring in labour

1. *Antepartum risk factors*:
   Primigravidae aged 35 or over; multigravidae aged 40 or over
   Grande multiparity
   Suspected IUGR
   Pregnancy-induced hypertension

History of APH in this pregnancy
Bad obstetric history
Diabetes
Multiple pregnancy
Rhesus iso-immunisation
Oligohydramnios
Reduced fetal movements
Abnormal antenatal FHR tracing or BPP

2. *Intrapartum risk factors*:
FHR >160 or <120 b.p.m.
Meconium-stained liquor
Prolonged labour
Epidural anaesthesia
Augmented labour
Pre-term labour
Supine hypotension
Breech presentation

Interpretation. The whole clinical situation must be considered.

Normal pattern
Rate between 120 and 160 b.p.m.
No significant change in rate during contractions
Baseline irregularity of ≥5 b.p.m.

Loss of baseline irregularity (<5 b.p.m.). This is the feature most commonly associated with fetal hypoxia. (Maternal drug administration can reduce baseline variability.) Management: check fetal pH.

Baseline bradycardia (FHR <120 b.p.m.). Only significant if it is accompanied by loss of baseline irregularity and/or decelerations (i.e. complicated bradycardia).
Management: turn the patient on her side, give oxygen and check fetal pH.

Baseline tachycardia (FHR >160 b.p.m.)
Management: measure fetal pH if tachycardia persists or it is accompanied by decelerations and/or loss of baseline irregularity.

Accelerations (at the start of a contraction returning to baseline). This is normal.

Early decelerations (Type 1 dip). A deceleration beginning with the onset of the contraction, returning to the baseline rate by the end of the contraction and usually <40 b.p.m. It may be due to head compression, cord compression or early hypoxia.
Management: check fetal pH if the pattern deteriorates.

Variable decelerations. A deceleration appearing at a variable time during the contraction, of irregular shape and >50 b.p.m. If they appear consistently, fetal hypoxia is likely.
Management: check fetal pH if the pattern persists after turning the patient on her side (or if other adverse features are present).

Late decelerations. A deceleration the lowest point of which is past the peak of the contraction. The greater the lag time the more serious the significance. The worst picture is of shallow late decelerations, loss of baseline irregularity and tachycardia.
Management: a fetal pH measurement is mandatory.
Dip area: a cumulative amplitude and duration of decelerations of more than 200 beats in any 20-minute period suggests hypoxia. Check fetal pH.

FHR in the second stage of labour
The fetal heart patterns are complex and difficult to interpret in the second stage of labour. Brief profound decelerations are not uncommon but prolonged bradycardia must not be ignored.

3. *Fetal blood sampling (FBS).*

FHR and scalp pH measurement are complementary. The former without the latter increases the Caesarean section rate unnecessarily because of false positive diagnoses.

The indications for FBS are outlined above.

Interpretation

pH >7.25	Normal	No action
pH 7.20–7.25	Borderline	Sample again in 30 minutes
pH <7.20	Abnormal	Deliver

See also the section on Methods of intrapartum monitoring (p. 129).

4. *Fetal ECG waveform.*

Change in the relationship between PR and R–R internals and the ST waveform may be a useful indicator of hypoxia. The main contribution is likely to be prevention of unnecessary Caesarean sections. For more details see Suggested further reading.

Significance of meconium staining of the liquor
Meconium is present in the liquor of about 15% of all deliveries at term and up to 40% post-term. It's significance as a diagnostic sign of 'fetal distress' has been over-emphasised although gross staining is more likely to be significant. Aspiration by the baby of the liquor heavily stained with meconium causes a severe and sometimes fatal pneumonitis. This should, therefore be avoided.

Conclusion
The sensitivity and specificity of methods for intrapartum monitoring of the fetus are still poor. New initiatives are still badly needed.

THE NORMAL PELVIS

Average diameters

	Diameters (cm)		
	Antero-posterior	Oblique	Transverse
Brim	11–11.5	12	12.5
Cavity	12	12	12
Outlet	12.5	12	11–11.5

Pelvic shape — in the normal pelvis
The *brim* is round, and the sacral promontory is not prominent. The angle of inclination is about 55° to the horizontal.
The *cavity* is shallow with straight, non-converging walls. The sacrum is smoothly curved.
In the outlet the sacro-sciatic notches are wide and shallow. The sacrum does not project forwards. The ischial spines are not prominent. The pubic arch is wide and domed. The sub-pubic angle is about 90°. The inter-tuberous diameter is wide accommodating four knuckles of the average-sized hand with ease.

X-ray pelvimetry
The lateral view is sufficient. The femoral head and acetabular margins must be superimposed (or very nearly so). The information to be gained is:
Relationship of presenting part to pelvic brim
Angle of inclination of the brim
Antero-posterior measurements of pelvic inlet, mid-pelvis and outlet
Discovery of false sacral promontory
Number of segments in the sacrum and its shape and angle
Width and depth of sacro-sciatic notches

Indications
Breech presentation at 37 weeks or later.

Postnatally after Caesarean section for suspected CPD (full pelvimetry possible here).

Previous Caesarean section when no pelvimetry has been performed.

CEPHALO-PELVIC DISPROPORTION (CPD)

Definition

The failure of the head to pass through the pelvis safely because the pelvis is too small and/or the head too large.

Diagnosis

CPD is more likely if maternal height is 1.5 metres or under.

1. Antenatally the fetal head cannot be made to engage by pressing it into the pelvic brim or with the patient standing
2. Labour fails to produce descent of the head and dilatation of the cervix but caput forms and excessive moulding occurs

Management

Elective section is seldom necessary in primigravidae unless:

1. There are other adverse features
2. There is a malpresentation
3. The true conjugate is <7.5 cm

Otherwise an attempt at vaginal delivery is justifiable. This is then regarded as a *trial of labour.*

A trial of labour should be allowed to continue for as long as progress is occurring in labour with regular forceful contractions. Progress is best monitored by the partogram. If the woman has not delivered within 12 hours of the onset of regular contractions the situation must be reviewed critically.

Such a trial of labour has no place in multigravid women or in the presence of a breech presentation.

ABNORMALITIES OF LIE, PRESENTATION AND POSITION

Breech presentation

Incidence

Two to three per cent of all labours. Up to one-third are undiagnosed.

Definition

Frank breech — (65%) both legs extended at the knee
Complete breech — (10%) both legs flexed at hip and knee
Footling breech — (25%) one or both feet tucked underneath the buttocks; more common in multiparous women due to laxity of abdomen

Causes
Extended legs preventing spontaneous version
Those conditions preventing the presenting part entering the pelvic cavity
Uterine anomaly
Chance

Associations
Fetal anomaly
Pre-term delivery
Multiple pregnancy

Antenatal management
External cephalic version (ECV) is safe for mother and baby in carefully selected patients and reduces the need to consider elective Caesarean section. Spontaneous version is likely up to 34 weeks. ECV can be attempted from 34 weeks using tocolytic agents as thought necessary. The use of general anaesthesia is totally unjustified.

Hazards of ECV
Pre-term labour
Abruptio placentae
Cord accident
Uterine rupture (if previous section)

Contra-indications to ECV

Absolute
- Multiple pregnancy
- APH
- Ruptured membranes
- Oligohydramnios
- Significant fetal anomaly
- Caesarean section indicated for other reasons

Relative
- Previous Caesarean section
- IUGR
- Hypertension
- Rhesus iso-immunisation
- Grande multiparity
- Anterior placenta
- Obesity

Rh-D-negative women must be given anti-D immunoglobulin (50 μmg or more as Kleihauer test dictates).

If the breech still presents at 37 weeks the size of the pelvis relative to the fetus and the fetal attitude should be assessed.

Management of delivery
It has been argued that breech presentation is indication enough for Caesarean section. Although vaginal breech delivery as a whole is associated with a higher perinatal mortality and morbidity than Caesarean section, these results are biased by the inclusion in the former group of very low birthweight infants for whom Caesarean section was not considered, or who delivered precipitately. The benefits of routine Caesarean section in both term and pre-term delivery have not been clearly demonstrated. A more conservative policy is outlined below.

Pre-delivery assessment
Pelvic dimensions clinically and radiologically at 37 weeks. Ultrasound assessment of BPD, fetal mass, fetal attitude and flexion/extension of fetal head. Major fetal anomalies should have been excluded

Vaginal delivery
An attempt at vaginal delivery can be considered with:
1. Term pregnancy and fetal weight estimated at 2500 to 3500 g
2. Frank breech
3. Normal pelvic dimensions
4. No other complications of pregnancy (e.g. pre-eclampsia)
5. Normal FHR tracing or biophysical profile

Epidural anaesthesia can be useful during a breech labour. Augmentation of labour with oxytocin is contra-indicated. The baby should be born by the patient's own efforts with little assistance from the obstetrician (assisted breech delivery). Any more active intervention involving breech extraction is contra-indicated because the perinatal consequences are so severe.

Caesarean section
Among the definite indications are:
Any abnormality of bony pelvis
Fetal weight estimated at >3.5 kg
Hyperextension of fetal head
Previous difficult labour
IUGR
Bad obstetric history
Older primigravidae
Diabetes
Severe pre-eclampsia
Failure to progress in first stage
Failure of descent of breech in second stage
Any condition which would apply whatever the presentation, e.g. fetal hypoxia

In the following, Caesarean section may be indicated. Any attempt at vaginal delivery must be clearly justified.
Complete or footling breech
Pre-term labour
Uterine anomaly
Pregnancy complications other than those noted above

Occipito-posterior position
If the baby's head is partially extended it does not fit into the lower uterine pole well, with the following consequences in labour:

1. The membranes rupture early and the cervix is not well apposed to the cervix
2. The sinciput reaches the pelvic floor first and therefore rotates to the front i.e. the occiput is posterior
3. The larger occipito-frontal diameter (10 cm) of the head presents, making its passage through the pelvis more difficult
4. The first stage of labour is prolonged
5. The moment of the forces pushes the head posteriorly causing backache and inducing bearing-down efforts before full dilatation
6. The second stage of labour may be prolonged

The occiput may:

1. Rotate anteriorly and deliver relatively easily (75%)
2. Persist posteriorly (POP) and delivery spontaneously if the pelvis is capacious (i.e. face to pubes) or require assisted delivery (5%)
3. Begin to rotate anteriorly but undergo deep transverse arrest at the level of the ischial spines. Instrumental delivery will be required (20%)

Predisposing factors
Slight reduction in pelvic inlet
Large baby

Diagnosis
Antenatally — the maternal abdomen may be flattened or fetal parts palpable easily on both sides of the midline. The head is unengaged and feels larger than usual.

Intrapartum — by vaginal examination: both fontanelles can be felt more easily. Moulding and caput may make recognition difficult and palpation of an ear may be necessary for correct positioning.

Management

1. Provide adequate analgesia: an epidural anaesthetic is ideal
2. Prevent maternal ketosis and dehydration
3. Observe progress in labour carefully

4. Monitor fetal welfare
5. Relative cephalo-pelvic disproportion may occur

The criteria for assisted delivery are discussed on p. 140.

Brow presentation

A brow presentation discovered antenatally may be due to: chance — and may correct itself spontaneously; a swelling in the neck causing extension of the head, e.g. goitre, cystic hygroma; spasm of the sterno-mastoid muscles.

Suspect a brow presentation in a multiparous woman with delay in the first stage of labour despite good contractions when she has delivered vaginally easily before.

Diagnosis

Supra-orbital ridges and anterior fontanelle palpatable p.v. Confirm by ultrasound.

Management

In early labour a brow presentation may flex to become a vertex or extend further to a face presentation. Both are potentially deliverable vaginally.

If the brow presentation persists into or is discovered in established labour, delivery should be by Caesarean section.

Face presentation

A face presentation has the same causes as a brow presentation but causing full extension of the head on the neck.

In labour anterior rotation of the chin is essential: a mento-posteror position cannot deliver vaginally.

Diagnosis

Palpation of supra-orbital ridges and the alveolar margins (confusion may arise between a face and the breech). X-ray will help to confirm.

Management

An attempt at vaginal delivery should be allowed unless:
1. Something is obstructing the entry into the pelvis
2. The pelvis is too small
3. The chin is posterior

Transverse and oblique lie

Causes

High multiparity
Pre-term labour
Multiple pregnancy
Uterine anomaly
Hydramnios

Obstructing tumour or placenta praevia
Severe pelvic contraction

Antenatal management (see p. 134)

Intrapartum management — (singleton pregnancy)
In a neglected shoulder presentation an arm may well be prolapsed and the baby already dead. In these circumstances vaginal decapitation may be possible but only by an experienced operator.

Otherwise Caesarean section with decapitation in utero is less hazardous for the mother.

MULTIPLE PREGNANCY AND LABOUR

Twins

Pre-term labour is common
Placenta praevia may be present
Prolapse of the cord must be watched for
Malpresentations are more likely — the presentations in order of frequency being:

1. Vertex: vertex
2. Vertex: breech
3. Breech: vertex
4. Breech: breech
5. Vertex: transverse
6. Breech: transverse

Possible indications for elective Caesarean section

First twin presenting as a breech
Pre-term labour (before 34 weeks)
Triplets (?) and higher multiples
Proteinuric pre-eclampsia
Any indication which would also apply in singleton pregnancies, e.g. IUGR, APH

Management of labour and delivery

An intravenous line should be set up and an anaesthetist should be present for delivery lest rapid general anaesthesia becomes necessary.

Once uterine activity begins the second sac should be ruptured. If contractions do not begin within 15 minutes commence an oxytocin infusion.

If the cord of the second twin is prolapsed proceed to ventouse extraction (if the presentation is cephalic) or breech extraction (if the presentation is breech). Anaesthesia for the latter should be epidural if already established, or general. The interval between delivery of the first and second twins should be no more than 20 minutes. Beware of postpartum haemorrhage.

After delivery check placentae and membranes for zygosity. Histological confirmation is necessary.

For triplets or quadruplets (and higher multiples) delivery by Caesarean section may be best although vaginal delivery of triplets can be achieved.

OPERATIVE OBSTETRICS

Episiotomy

The need for an episiotomy is a matter for experienced clinical judgement. It should never be carried out merely because 'it is routine'.

Indications

Among these will be:

1. When a perineal tear appears inevitable otherwise
2. In cases of fetal distress late in the second stage
3. Most forceps deliveries (except low cavity forceps)
4. Pre-term delivery
5. Breech delivery
6. Failure to advance because of perineal rigidity.

Too many episiotomies are performed in modern obstetrics and there is little evidence that the number of vaginal lacerations is reduced.

Technique

An episiotomy must be:

1. Performed at the correct time — incise too early and unnecessary blood loss will result
2. Carried out with adequate local or regional anaesthesia. Failure to use anaesthesia is to be deprecated
3. Made with sharp scissors in the correct place. The medio-lateral episiotomy is more common in the UK but the risks of the midline incision have been exaggerated. The episiotomy must always start in the midline
4. Repaired properly within as short a time of delivery as possible

Side-effects

Pain. This can be severe and is the main reason for avoiding episiotomy. It can be reduced by prompt, careful and expert repair.

Bleeding. The average blood loss is about 100 ml and much larger losses are all too common.

Breakdown. Inversely related to the expertise of the person repairing the episiotomy. Potential causes are delay in suturing, inappropriate suture materials, bad technique, too much catgut left in the wound, too tight sutures.

Dyspareunia. This can be severe and can be one factor in ultimate marital breakdown.

Third degree tear

Definition
When a vaginal laceration or episiotomy extends to involve at least the anal mucosa.

They must be repaired in theatre under epidural or general anaesthesia by an experienced obstetrician. The rectum then the anus are first repaired with interrupted catgut sutures (knots towards the gut lumen). If necessary the vagina and rectum should be dissected apart in the upper part of the tear. The torn ends of the sphincter are then localised and sutured. The residual second degree tear is repaired routinely.

After-care
Low residue diet for one week followed by high bulk diet.
Normacol to soften the faeces.
If the repair breaks down eradicate local sepsis before attempting another repair.

Instrumental delivery

Potential indications

1. Failure to advance in the second stage, frequently due to failure of maternal effort, epidural analgesia and/or malposition of the fetal head
2. Maternal conditions in which (prolonged) expulsive efforts may be detrimental e.g. cardiac and respiratory disease, severe pre-eclampsia or eclampsia
3. 'Fetal distress' in the second stage
4. Prolapse of the cord in the second stage

Delivery can be by obstetric forceps or the vacuum extractor (ventouse).

Prior conditions for the proper use of forceps

1. A legitimate indication must be present
2. The presentation must be suitable i.e. vertex, face (mento-anterior) or after-coming head in a breech delivery
3. There must be no cephalo-pelvic disproportion. Moulding of the fetal skull must not be excessive
4. The head must be engaged. Ideally no part of the fetal head should be palpable per abdomen, and if more than 1/5 can be palpated vaginal delivery must not be contemplated
5. The position of the head must be known
6. The cervix must be fully dilated
7. Analgesia must be adequate

8. The bladder must be empty
9. The uterus must be contracting

The same conditions apply to the proper use of the ventouse except that it may be used before the cervix has reached full dilatation. The ventouse must not be considered as an easy way out when adverse features are present or the position of the fetal head is unknown.

Face-to-pubes delivery with forceps

In certain cases it may be preferable to deliver the head with the occiput still posterior. This requires great judgement and must be carried out with even greater care.

Potential indications

1. The head is directly occipito-posterior (OP) and low in the pelvis
2. The pelvis has a narrow transverse diameter inhibiting rotation but still allowing safe delivery

Forceps to the after-coming head (ACH) in a breech delivery

This is the method of choice for delivery of the ACH because of the degree of control the operator can exercise.

Forceps in the delivery of low birthweight infants (<2500 g)

The use of forceps in pre-term delivery and for other low birthweight (LBW) infants is based on the false premise that the forceps protect against intraventricular haemorrhage. This is, however, *not* caused by trauma but is related to prolonged hypoxia particularly in RDS. Lift-out forceps neither protects against nor induces birth trauma in LBW infants. Their use is therefore optional. Rotational forceps are more dangerous for LBW infants and they must be used judiciously if at all.

Trial of forceps

This is justifiable when it is likely, but not entirely certain, that vaginal delivery by forceps will be successful. Otherwise the patient should be delivered by Caesarean section. It should be carried out in a theatre fully prepared for Caesarean section.

The use of the ventouse

Vaginal delivery is said to be feasible from 5 cm. The following points are a guide to its proper use:

1. The patient's expulsive efforts are used to assist delivery
2. The fetal head must be at least at the level of the spines
3. The largest possible of the four cups should be used
4. If delivery is not imminent after pulling on the ventouse during three contractions the attempt must cease and the patient must be delivered by Caesarean section

Analgesia for instrumental delivery
Perineal infiltration alone is suitable for episiotomy, and low outlet deliveries using Wrigley's forceps or the ventouse.
Pudendal nerve block is useful for mid-cavity forceps and some ventouse deliveries. It does not provide adequate analgesia for rotational forceps. The transvaginal route is recommended for insertion of the block.
Epidural anaesthesia is ideal particularly for rotational forceps; it is also suitable for elective Caesarean sections and those emergency sections in which an existing epidural block is providing good analgesia.
General anaesthesia may be necessary for some rotational forceps e.g. if there is 'fetal distress' and no time to insert an epidural block.

Caesarean section
This procedure must not be carried out without good reasons. It is indicated when delivery must be effected rapidly for fetal and/or maternal reasons and this is not possible safely vaginally.
The transperitoneal lower segment Caesarean section accounts for virtually all of the operations in modern obstetrics.
Classical Caesarean section is very occasionally indicated e.g. for transverse lie with PROM, or for Caesarean section at 26 to 28 weeks. In this latter situation the vertical incision starts in the lower segment but extends into the upper segment.

Epidural anaesthesia and Caesarean section
Advantages
The mother is awake and sees the child at delivery.
The father can usually be present.
Consciousness is not impaired immediately postoperatively.
Postoperative problems and pain are less than after general anaesthesia.
Breast feeding and mobilisation can start early.

Disadvantages
The procedure takes longer.
Sometimes anaesthesia is not complete (the patient should be fully prepared for general anaesthesia).
Contra-indications to epidural anaesthesia are discussed on p. 125.

Some important technical points about LSCS
1. Antacids should be given pre-operatively to reduce the risk from aspiration of acid gastric contents
2. Induction of anaesthesia should take place of the last possible moment to reduce fetal exposure to the anaesthetic agents

3. The operation is carried out with a 10 to 15 degree left lateral tilt to prevent supine hypotension
4. A cuffed endotracheal tube must be used
5. Special care must be taken in Rh-negative women to remove residual blood from the peritoneal cavity because some of it may be Rh D-positive fetal blood
6. Early ambulation is encouraged to reduce the risk of thrombo-embolism
7. Operation should not prevent early breast-feeding
8. Carry out X-ray pelvimetry in the puerperium if vaginal delivery is contemplated in subsequent pregnancies

Delivery in subsequent pregnancies
Elective Caesarean section is necessary:
1. If the cause is recurrent, e.g. CPD
2. If pelvic dimensions are reduced

If vaginal delivery is attempted:
Oxytocin must be used only with the strongest of indications; it is helpful to monitor intrauterine pressures in this situation.
Epidural anaesthesia can be used; the pain of ruptured uterus will break through the epidural block.
The integrity of the lower segment must be checked after the baby is delivered.

Maternal mortality and Caesarean section
There were 69 maternal deaths due to Caesarean section in England and Wales in the years 1982–84 (i.e. 0.4 deaths/1000 Caesarean sections). Of these, 44 were directly related to the operation, and over half were associated with avoidable factors. The main associated causes of death (in order) were:

Pulmonary embolus	(17%)
Hypertensive complications	(14%)
Anaesthetic complications	(12%)

Sepsis was associated with only 1 death.

Inhalation of stomach contents (Mendelson's syndrome)
This accounts for 50% of obstetric anaesthetic deaths.

Prevention
All labouring women should be given oral sodium citrate as an antacid. For elective Caesarean section (whether under general anaesthesia or by epidural) inhibit gastric acid secretions with H_2 antagonists (e.g. ranitidine) and give sodium citrate. For emergency Caesarean section give i.v. ranitidine and oral sodium citrate when the decision to proceed is made, and repeat the sodium citrate just before induction of anaesthesia.
Clinical presentation — cyanosis, tachycardia, bronchospasm, pulmonary oedema, deepening shock in relation to general anaesthesia. It may be confused with pulmonary oedema

secondary to mitral stenosis, cardiac failure or amniotic fluid embolism.

Management

1. Tilt the patient's head down
2. Turn her on one side and aspirate the pharynx
3. Give oxygen
4. Inject aminophylline and hydrocortisone i.v. and repeat as necessary
5. Suck bronchial tree clear through a bronchoscope (under GA)
6. Prescribe broad-spectrum antibiotics

SUGGESTED FURTHER READING

Beard R W, Sharp F (eds) 1985 Preterm labour and its consequences. Proceedings of the thirteenth study group of the RCOG

Enkin M, Keirse M, Chalmers I 1989 Effective care in pregnancy and childbirth. Oxford University Press, Oxford

Greene K R 1987 The ECG waveform. Clinical Obstetrics and Gynaecology 1: 131–155

O'Driscoll K, Meagher D 1986 Active management of labour. 2nd edn. Saunders, London

Stirrat G M 1986 Pocket consultant in obstetrics, 2nd edn. Blackwell, Oxford

Turnbull A, Chamberlain G (eds) 1989 Obstetrics. Churchill Livingstone, Edinburgh

Third-stage problems and obstetric emergencies

THE NORMAL THIRD STAGE OF LABOUR

This begins with delivery of the baby and ends with expulsion of the placenta.

Management

'Physiological' management of the third stage involves:

1. Division of the umbilical cord only when pulsation has ceased
2. Delivery of the placenta by maternal effort and aided by gravity without cord traction
3. Use of oxytocics only if haemorrhage occurs

This policy allows blood volume to equilibrate between mother and baby and avoids side-effects of oxytocin.

'Active' management of the third stage has become routine over the past 20 years in the UK and has recently been shown to be associated with reduced blood loss overall. This involves:

1. Syntometrine (syntocinon 5 units: ergometrine 0.5 mg) with delivery of the anterior shoulder
2. Delivery of the placenta by *controlled cord traction* (CCT) when separation has occurred

POSTPARTUM HAEMORRHAGE AND RETAINED PLACENTA

Definition

Primary postpartum haemorrhage is the loss of 500 ml or more of blood within 24 hours of delivery.

Incidence

It accounted for 3 maternal deaths in England and Wales between 1982 and 1984.

The incidence varies from 2 to 8% among hospitals.

Associated factors

1. Grande multiparity (associated with uterine atony)

2. Delivery after an APH (due to placenta praevia or abruptio placentae)
3. Multiple pregnancy
4. Polyhydramnios
5. Past history of PPH
6. Coagulative disorders

Main causes

1. Retained placenta (in part or whole)
2. Uterine atony
3. Soft tissue lacerations
4. Defective coagulation

Management

Prevention

Proper management of the third stage, e.g. do not 'fiddle' with the uterine fundus while waiting for placental separation.

Treatment

1. Rub up a uterine contraction
2. Correct hypovolaemia by intravenous fluids and screened Group O Rh-D negative, Kell-negative blood if necessary
3. Remove the placenta if it is retained or incomplete using general or epidural anaesthesia. Basal narcosis (pethidine 50 mg and diazepam 100 mg i.v.) may be used in extreme situations
4. Check for vaginal, cervical or uterine lacerations
5. Maintain uterine contraction with an oxytocin infusion
6. Deal with coagulation failure as described on p. 149

Management of massive haemorrhage (see Report on Confidential Enquiries into Maternal Deaths in England and Wales 1982–84)

Prompt action is necessary:

1. Summon all extra staff required — obstetricians, anaesthetists, midwives, porters (to relay samples and fetch blood). Alert haematologist and blood transfusion service
2. Set up at least two large infusion lines
3. Monitor CVP, intra-arterial pressure, heart rate, ECG, pO_2, and urine output
4. Send at least 20 ml of blood for cross-matching and coagulation screen. Order a minimum of 6 units of blood
5. Give warmed whole blood if possible (under pressure if necessary) but if only plasma reduced blood is available infuse additional colloid if more than 3 units are given. Do not give FFP or platelets until haemorrhage has stopped or at least 5 units of stored blood have been given. Avoid dextran. The primary aim is to restore circulating volume

6. Internal iliac ligation and/or hysterectomy are rarely necessary. If indicated, laparotomy must be embarked on before the situation is desperate

Morbid adherence of the placenta (placenta accreta)
This is a rare occurrence. As much of the placenta as possible should be removed manually under GA and the uterus packed. Transfusion will be necessary.

Severe degrees of placenta accreta will require hysterectomy.

CORD PRESENTATION AND PROLAPSE

Cord presentation discovered before rupture of the membranes is an indication for immediate Caesarean section.
Cord prolapse is associated with all factors maintaining the presenting part high above the pelvis or when it does not fit well into the pelvis at the time of rupture of the membranes, e.g. transverse lie, polyhydramnios, CPD, pre-term labour, multiple pregnancy or breech presentation.
Diagnosis — the cord is visible or palpable. Consider the diagnosis if fetal distress occurs in association with spontaneous rupture of the membranes.

Management depends on whether or not the child is alive. If it is, and the cervix is fully dilated, expedite delivery with forceps (or breech extraction perhaps).

If the cervix is not fully dilated arrange urgent Caesarean section.

Emergency procedures
1. Displace the presenting part with the examining hand
2. Fill the bladder with 750 ml of normal saline by indwelling catheter
3. Drop the end of the bed or stretcher
4. Keep the patient in the knee–elbow position until delivery can be effected

UTERINE RUPTURE

Uterine rupture caused 3 maternal deaths in England and Wales between 1982 and 1984. Main associated factors:
1. Previous Caesarean section scar (often classical)
2. The inappropriate use of oxytocin to augment labour (e.g. in multiparous women)
3. Previous cervical surgery
4. Failure to recognise obstructed labour

Signs and symptoms
Severe bursting pain (which will even break through an epidural

block). However, she may only complain of some lower abdominal discomfort
Unexplained tachycardia
Variable amounts of vaginal bleeding
Fainting and ensuing shock
Cessation of contractions
Disappearance of the presenting part from the pelvis
Fetal distress
The possibility of an unrecognised rupture must be considered when bleeding continues after delivery despite well-retracted uterus, or there is unexplained shock (particularly if she was delivered by forceps or has had a previous Caesarean section).

Management

1. Arrange immediate laparotomy
2. Transfuse
3. Carry out the least extensive surgery compatible with the patient's immediate health and future welfare
4. Take great care to identify the ureters and exclude them from any sutures
5. If hysterectomy is not carried out consider tubal ligation

Future pregnancies

Close observation is required during any future pregnancy, and delivery should be by elective Caesarean section at 38 weeks.

UTERINE INVERSION

This is a profoundly shocking complication. It is often caused by injudicious cord traction with an atonic uterus when the insertion of the placenta is fundal.

The inversion may not be complete and therefore not immediately visible. Diagnosis is by vaginal examination.

Management

1. Try to reduce the inversion
2. Initiate anti-shock measures
3. If the placenta is still attached and easily removable, do so, once the shock has been corrected
4. The hydrostatic method for reduction is usually effective:
   (i) The inverted uterus is held within the vagina
   (ii) Two litres of warm saline are infused rapidly into the vagina and the even hydrostatic pressure exerted usually reduces the inverted uterus

For further details see: Stirrat, in Suggested further reading.

AMNIOTIC FLUID EMBOLISM

This caused 14 maternal deaths between 1982 and 1984 in England and Wales plus another 2 suspected cases.

Associated factors

Precipitate labour
Polyhydramnios
Hypertonic uterine action (with or without oxytocin)
Induction or augmentation of labour with prostaglandin pessaries

Signs and symptoms

1. Profound shock
2. Cyanosis
3. Dyspnoea
4. Severe coagulation defect

Management

1. Prevent death from pulmonary vascular obstruction: oxygen; hydrocortisone; endotracheal intubation
2. Control coagulation defect

COAGULATION FAILURE

Main causes in pregnancy

Placental abruption
Amniotic fluid embolism
Endotoxic shock

Diagnosis

Clinical observation
Whole blood clotting time (normal 5 to 10 minutes)
Thrombin clotting time — a sample of blood added to a tube containing a small amount of thrombin should clot within 10 seconds
Reduction in platelet count
Reduced fibrinogen titres
Increased levels of fibrin degradation products

Management

1. The coagulation defect is usually self-limiting if the stimulus producing it is removed. Therefore the uterus should be emptied as expeditiously as possible
2. Transfuse, using fresh blood — see Management of massive haemorrhage (p. 146)

ACUTE ABDOMINAL PAIN IN PREGNANCY

The differential diagnosis of acute abdominal pain can be difficult in pregnancy.

Causes incidental to pregnancy
For example:
Appendicitis
Accident to ovarian cyst
Acute cholecystitis
Renal calculus
Intestinal obstruction
Volvulus
Perforated peptic ulcer
Rectus abdominis haematoma

Causes related to pregnancy

Early pregnancy
Abortion (including septic)
Cornual pregnancy (or other ectopic pregnancy)
Acute retention of urine due to retroverted gravid uterus

Later pregnancy
Abruptio placentae
Uterine rupture
Severe pre-eclampsia
Degeneration of fibroid
Pyelonephritis
Extrauterine pregnancy
Appendicitis can be difficult to diagnose in pregnancy because:
1. The appendix is displaced upward
2. The site of pain is often atypical
3. Examination is made difficult by the pregnant uterus
4. The body's reaction (e.g. leucocytosis) may be masked

SUGGESTED FURTHER READING

Baskett T F 1985 Essential management of obstetric emergencies. Wiley, Chichester
Enkin M, Keirse M J N C, Chalmers I 1989 Effective care in pregnancy and childbirth. Oxford University Press, Oxford
Reports–Confidential Enquiries into Maternal Deaths in England & Wales 1982–84. 1989 HMSO, London
Stirrat G M 1986 An obstetric pocket consultant. Blackwell, Oxford
Turnbull A, Chamberlain G (eds) 1989 Obstetrics. Churchill Livingstone, Edinburgh

Perinatal and maternal mortality

DEFINITIONS

Livebirth

The complete expulsion or extraction from its mother of a product of conception, irrespective of gestational age, which then breathes or shows any evidence of life such as beating of the heart, pulsation of the umbilical cord, or definite movement of voluntary muscles.

Stillbirth

Birth of an infant who shows no evidence of life after birth.

Death, fetal (prenatal death)

Death of a fetus *in utero* which, at birth, weighs 500 g or more irrespective of gestational age.

Death, infant, early neonatal

Death of a liveborn infant occurring less than 7 completed days (168 hours) from the time of birth.

Death, infant, late neonatal

Death of a liveborn infant after 7 completed days of age but before 28 completed days.

The perinatal period

Commences when a fetus has developed to a weight of 1000 g (approximately equivalent to 28 weeks' gestation); it ends when the newborn baby has achieved an age of 7 completed days (168 hours) of life. In the absence of measured birthweight, a body length of 35 cm is considered equivalent to 1000 g birthweight. When neither birthweight nor body length has been measured, a fetus is considered to have entered the perinatal period when the gestational age has reached 28 completed weeks (196 days).

PERINATAL MORTALITY

The perinatal mortality rate (PMR) is the number of stillbirths and first-week deaths occurring from 28 completed weeks of pregnancy to seven days after birth per 1000 total births.

Confusions

If an infant is born before 28 weeks' gestation and shows signs of life but then dies within 7 days it is to be included as a perinatal death. Some countries include births from 20 weeks' gestation and deaths up to 28 days postpartum.

Recommendations (Ninth Revision of ICD, WHO, 1980)

1. National perinatal statistics should include infants with birthweight > 500 g *or* at least 22 completed weeks *or* crown–heel length at least 25 cm
2. For international statistics the minima should be birthweight 1000 g, gestational age 28 weeks or crown–heel length 35 cm

PMR in England and Wales (per 1000 total births)

1931–35	62.5
1961–65	29.4
1976–78	16.7
1983	10.4
1988	8.7 (range 6.7–10.3)

Factors influencing PMR

Birthweight

PMR and birthweight are closely related. Comparison of rates among populations must be broken down by birthweight groups.

Although infants < 2500 g comprise only 7% of all births, 50% of all perinatal and infant deaths occurred in this group. The mortality among infants < 1500 g is almost 50%. Above 1500 g mortality rates fall dramatically as birthweight increases. The lowest rate occurs over 3000 g.

Social class and legitimacy

Perinatal mortality rises as social class falls.

Perinatal mortality 1986 in England and Wales

Total	9.5/1000 total births
Legitimate births	8.8
Social class I and II	7.2
Social class V	11.4
Illegitimate births	12.3

Maternal age and parity
The PMR is at its lowest in mothers between the ages of 25 and 29 years and for the second child. It increases three-fold for mothers aged 40 to 44, doubles for the fifth child, and trebles for the seventh. This is influenced by social class and the association of congenital anomalies with age.

Race
The PMR is raised among immigrants from Pakistan, East and West Africa and the West Indies.

Multiple births

Smoking

Perinatal mortality rates
Perinatal mortality rates are commonly used as an indicator of standards of obstetric care. This is inappropriate for the following reasons:

1. International comparisons are confounded by different definitions
2. In the developed world perinatal death is no longer common enough to allow it to be used in this way. In the developing world data collection is incomplete
3. Sixty per cent of the deaths remain unexplained and are not associated with any risk marker
4. Two of the major contributors, lethal congenital malformations and very pre-term delivery, are not influenced by obstetric care in that they cannot truly be prevented by it
5. Up to 25% of the decline in PNM can be explained by increases in birthweight due to socio-economic changes
6. Much of the remaining decline is due to improvements in neonatal rather than obstetric care

PERINATAL MORBIDITY

There are no national statistics available for perinatal morbidity or subsequent disability, neither is there any agreed definition of disability. It is not at all clear that the incidence of disability will fall as mortality is reduced.

It is still not clear what factors affect the developmental achievements of children and why one child suffers while another does not.

PERINATAL PATHOLOGY

A good perinatal pathology service is fundamental to the practice of modern obstetrics. Perinatal pathology services should be established on a regional basis.

The following are among the procedures which must be undertaken in the event of a perinatal death:

1. *Detailed inspection and measurement of the baby* (minimum requirements). Measure weight, crown–heel, crown–rump, and foot lengths, occipito-frontal circumference. Look for malformations, deformations, state of maceration (if any) and evidence of trauma. Pay special attention to limbs, genitalia and facies
2. *Detailed clinical information must be supplied to the pathologist* (preferably on a structured request form), who should also have access to the case notes
3. *Request an autopsy* in all cases, even when the cause seems obvious. Autopsy rates under 75% are unacceptable. In the case of stillbirth, submit fetus and placenta together. The placenta of every baby born weighing less than 1500 g and/or less than the third centile for gestational age and sex, and of all multiple pregnancies, should be sent for examination because these babies are at greatest risk of neonatal death
4. *Maternal investigations* are the responsibility of the obstetrician. These should include (as a minimum): TORCH screen, Kleihauer test, VDRL and Rh or other antibodies if not checked antenatally, random blood sugar and glycosylated Hb or fructosamine
5. *The extent of the further investigation* of the baby depends on the autopsy findings, measurements and histological examination (of baby and placenta). These are the guide to further cytogenetic, biochemical, microbiological or haematological investigations required. If dwarfism is suspected X-ray examination is mandatory
6. The parents must be treated with the utmost compassion and be encouraged (but not forced) to see their dead child even if disfiguring abnormalities are present. A polaroid photograph should be taken and kept for the parents to see and keep when they wish. Informed assistance should be given with registration and funeral arrangements. The GP and community midwife must be informed quickly
7. The couple should be seen by the obstetrician (and paediatrician in the case of a NND) when all the information on the case is available

MATERNAL MORTALITY

Definition

The death of the mother occurring during pregnancy or labour, or as a consequence of pregnancy within 42 days of delivery or abortion.

Deaths are considered as (a) directly attributable to pregnancy

— *direct deaths*, or (b) resulting from a condition which preceded or developed during pregnancy the effect of which was aggravated by the pregnancy — *indirect deaths*.

The maternal mortality rate is expressed per million 'maternities', i.e. pregnancy, childbirth or abortion.

Main direct causes of maternal deaths in England and Wales 1976–1984 (per million maternities)

	1976–78	*1979–81*	*1982–84*
Hypertensive diseases of pregnancy	12.5	14.2	10.0
Pulmonary embolism	18.5	9.0	10.0
Anaesthesia	11.6	8.7	7.2
Amniotic fluid embolism	4.7	7.1	5.6
Abortion	6.0	5.5	4.4
Ectopic pregnancy	9.0	7.9	4.0
Haemorrhage	10.3	5.5	3.6
Ruptured uterus	6.0	1.6	1.2
Sepsis (excluding abortion and ectopic pregnancy)	6.5	3.1	0.8
Miscellaneous causes	8.2	7.5	8.4
Overall rate	93.4	70.0	55.0

Many deaths are still associated with substandard care.

SUGGESTED FURTHER READING

Confidential enquiry into maternal mortality in England and Wales 1982–84, HMSO (and continuing triennial series)

Turnbull A, Chamberlain G 1989 Obstetrics. Churchill Livingstone, Edinburgh

The puerperium

The puerperium is the period of time over which the genital tract returns to normal after childbirth. It is taken as lasting for 6 weeks.

THE NORMAL PUERPERIUM

It is characterised by:
Lactation
Lochia
Involution of the uterus and return of the genital tract to normal

Suppression of lactation

This is seldom necessary. Bromocriptine can be used.

Management of engorgement

1. Firm support of breasts with a good bra
2. Adequate analgesia
3. Warm bathing of breasts
4. Expression should be avoided
5. If needs be bromocriptine can be prescribed

PUERPERAL PYREXIA

Definition

Temperature of 38°C on any occasion in the first 14 days after delivery or miscarriage (a slight fever is not uncommon within the first 24 hours after delivery).

Causes

Urinary tract infection
Genital tract infection
Breast infection
Deep vein thrombosis
Respiratory infection

Other non-obstetric causes
Intrauterine infection

Investigation
Full clinical investigation (including breasts and legs)
MSU
Cervical and high vaginal swabs
Blood culture
Sputum culture (if possible)

Management
After the investigations have been sent to the laboratory, and if the clinical situation warrants it, antibiotic therapy can be started.

Mastitis
Acute intramammary mastitis is due to failure of milk withdrawal from a lobule. Treatment involves getting the baby to empty the breast, cold compresses, and antibiotics if there is no improvement within 24 hours.
Infective mastitis may be due to *Staph. aureus*, and treatment with an antibiotic to which that organism is sensitive may be necessary.
Breast abscess formation is rare but preventable. Antibiotics are of value only if given early. An established abscess requires surgical drainage.

SECONDARY POSTPARTUM HAEMORRHAGE

Definition
Excessive blood loss from the genital tract for more than 24 hours and within 6 weeks of delivery. The amount is not specified.

Causes

Retained placental fragments	}	usually within a few days
Blood clot		of delivery

Management
If the bleeding has been slight and there is no evidence of infection the patient needs no more than to be kept under observation. Treatment with oral ergometrine is of doubtful value.

Careful evacuation of the uterus under general anaesthesia is indicated if:
An ultrasound scan suggests the presence of retained products
Heavy bleeding persists
The uterus is larger than expected and tender; the cervix is open. Infection is treated appropriately

PERINEAL PAIN

Prevention

Avoidance of trauma at delivery, and proper repair of tears or episiotomy.

Treatment

1. Local anaesthetic sprays relieve pain in the immediate postpartum period. There is no evidence that ice, salt or other baths, or herbal remedies, produce lasting benefit. Local steroids should be avoided
2. Relief of pressure on perineum
3. Ultrasound or pulsed electromagnetic energy — controlled trials show no clear benefit
4. Analgesia — paracetemol or NSAIDs for mild pain; unfortunately no analgesic seems to be of value for severe pain

EFFECTS OF CHILDBIRTH ON PELVIC FLOOR MUSCLES AND NERVES

The pelvic floor muscles and nerves are damaged even by a normal delivery. Ventouse extraction is usually less traumatic than forceps. Obstetric trauma predisposes to faecal incontinence. Division of the external anal sphincter at delivery is associated with long-term and sometimes severe effects on anal canal sensation and function.

SUGGESTED FURTHER READING

Dunlop W 1989 The puerperium. Fetal Medicine Review 1: 43–60
Turnbull A, Chamberlain G 1989 Obstetrics. Churchill Livingstone, Edinburgh

The newborn infant

ASSESSMENT AT BIRTH

Apgar score

This should be carried out on all babies at 1 and 5 minutes after birth. Scores of nought to two are given for each of the following parameters:

1. Heart rate
2. Respiratory effort
3. Muscle tone
4. Response to catheter in nostril
5. Colour

A score of seven or less at 5 minutes suggests some degree of birth asphyxia.

Routine examination within 2 hours of birth. The object of the examination is to ask:

1. Is the baby pre-term or small-for-dates?
2. Are cyanosis, jaundice or anaemia apparent?
3. Is there evidence of birth trauma?
4. Are there any congenital anomalies?

Assessment of gestational age

Gestational age can be assessed independently of knowledge of menstrual age using a score from a series of physical criteria (the Farr Score) which can be used alone or in combination with an assessment of neurological criteria (Dubowicz score). The total score can be translated into an estimate of gestational age. For further information see Stirrat, in Suggested further reading.

RESUSCITATION

The priorities of resuscitation are:

1. Maintenance of body temperature
2. Clearance of airways
3. Establishment of ventilation (with or without administration of oxygen)

Indication for the presence of neonatal paediatrician (or equivalent) at delivery

All Caesarean sections
All instrumental deliveries
Pre-term delivery
IUGR
APH
Polyhydramnios
Multiple pregnancy
Maternal history of diabetes, ITP, myasthenia, thyrotoxicosis, drug abuse
Fetal anomaly
Suspected amnionitis
Breech delivery
Meconium staining of liquor
Severe rhesus-isoimmunisation

Admission to special care baby unit (SCBU)

Babies should not be separated from their mothers without good cause. The following babies usually need further special care on SCBU or transitional care ward:

1. After prolonged resuscitation
2. Birth weight less than 2000 g
3. Gestational age less than 36 weeks
4. Persisting respiratory problem
5. Some severe congenital anomalies
6. All ill babies
7. Infants of drug-abusing mothers

The mother and father should be given an opportunity to see and hold the baby before transfer if at all possible.

NEONATAL SCREENING AND TREATMENT

Phenylketonuria (PKU)

The incidence is 1 in 10 000 live births. The Guthrie test or a chromatographic test should be carried out routinely within 7 to 14 days of delivery. If the Guthrie bacteriological test is used it should be postponed if the baby is on antibiotics.

Congenital hypothyroidism

The incidence is about 1 in 4000 live births. Without a screening programme for its detection only 40% of cases will be diagnosed by 3 months of age. Hypothyroidism can lead to mental retardation unless treated early. Testing (on a dried blood filter-paper spot) can be carried out at the same time as for PKU. TSH alone or T_4 and TSH are measured.

Congenital dislocation of the hip

If the hips are or can be dislocated, treat in an abduction splint (for 8–12 weeks) and refer to a paediatrician or orthopaedic surgeon.

BCG vaccination

BCG should be given to:

1. Newborn children in families known to have had tuberculosis whatever the type and however long ago
2. Children of *all* Asian immigrant families (tuberculosis is still widespread in the Asian communities amongst those who have been in the country for some years)
3. If the mother's sputum is positive for tuberculosis the baby should be given isoniazid-resistant BCG and treated with isoniazid. Baby and mother should be kept separate until the mother has been on anti-tuberculous treatment for 2 weeks

Ophthalmia neonatorum

Definition
Any purulent discharge from the eyes of an infant starting within 21 days of birth. It is still a notifiable disease and can cause severe damage if not treated promptly and adequately.

Causes
1. *Neisseria gonorrhoeae*
2. Other bacteria
3. *Chlamydia trachomatis*

Treatment should be in consultation with an ophthalmologist and venereologist.

Neonatal jaundice

If a term baby becomes jaundiced note date of onset, method of feeding, maternal blood group, history of perinatal trauma, and use of large volume of syntocinon containing fluid during labour.

Bilirubin level $> 200\ \mu$mol/l within 48 hours of birth needs prompt investigation, e.g.:
1. Proportion of direct bilirubin in blood
2. Blood group of mother and baby
3. Coombs' test and other antibodies
4. FBC, reticulocytes and differential white cell count
5. Urine for microscopy and reducing substances
6. Thyroid function tests
7. Glucose-6-phosphate dehydrogenase assay

Phototherapy will reduce the level and extent of the jaundice. It disrupts contact between baby and parents who may find it distressing. It is of no proven value for term infants over 48 hours of age with bilirubin levels $< 300\ \mu$mol/l.

DISCHARGE EXAMINATION

All babies should be examined in the presence of the mother before going home in order to:
1. Assess his or her progress from birth
2. Exclude malformations or traumatic lesions missed earlier

3. Identify any superficial infections
4. Reassure the mother

The following should be checked:

1. Baby's general appearance
2. Superficial infections (and other lesions) for eyes, mouth, umbilicus, nails
3. Heart for murmurs
4. Abdomen (NB The liver is normally 1 to 2 cm palpable)
5. Male genitalia for hypospadias, undescended testes, herniae and hydrocoeles
6. Female genitalia for vaginal discharge, fused labia, enlarged clitoris
7. Hips for congenital dislocation } discuss with orthopaedic
8. Feet for talipes equino varus } surgeon if present

SUGGESTED FURTHER READING

Fleming P J, Speidel B D, Dunn P M 1990 A neonatal vade mecum, 2nd edn. Lloyd-Luke, London

Obstetrics in the Third World

Childbirth is still the main cause of death of females of reproductive age in the developing world.

Probably more than 90% of pregnant women throughout the world deliver without having ever been in contact with anyone formally trained in any form of obstetric care.

Antenatal, intrapartum and postpartum care is supervised by the traditional birth attendant all too often in the context of malnutrition, infection and unregulated fertility. Even uncontaminated water is unavailable for the majority of the world's pregnant women.

Even when lack of care is not due to ignorance, bad communication and lack of transport make contact with a clinic or hospital impossible, particularly during heavy rains or other severe climatic conditions.

Among the particular problems which affect even those fortunate enough to have access to the most basic care are:

1. Illegal abortion
2. Trophoblastic tumours (particularly Latin America, Far East and Eastern Asia)
3. Severe anaemia
4. Malaria
5. HIV, hepatitis and other infections (particularly STDs)
6. Pre-eclampsia and eclampsia
7. Antepartum and postpartum haemorrhage
8. Obstructed labour (resulting in rupture of the uterus, stillbirth and/or obstetric fistulae)
9. Sepsis

The incidence of low birthweight is high due both to pre-term labour and IUGR.

MATERNAL MORTALITY IN THE THIRD WORLD

WHO reports overall maternal mortality rates (MMR) in Third World countries of between 1 and 4 per 1000 births rising to 78 per 1000 among unbooked patients in Indonesia (cf. UK < 0.1 per 1000 births).

The main causes overall are abortion, anaemia, eclampsia, haemorrhage, sepsis, and obstructed labour and its consequences.

PERINATAL MORTALITY IN THE THIRD WORLD

Perinatal mortality rates (PMR) are said to range from 35 to 80/1000 births, but in most Third World countries the true picture is unknown.

Infection is the main perinatal hazard, particularly in low-birthweight babies. However, among the other main causes are intrapartum asphyxia, meconium aspiration, pre-eclampsia and syphilis.

Traditional practices account for the high incidence of tetanus neonatorum.

REMEDIES

Western-style medicine is inappropriate because its high cost technology cannot be properly maintained and it takes finances away from more locally appropriate care. Socio-economic remedies are paramount, with improved fertility control and greater status for women in society. A hospital-based programme of obstetric care is beyond reach of every developing country and is not appropriate for any but high-risk patients. Thus, when services are planned they must be practical (i.e. achievable now) and form a basis for future development and extension.

The only possible basis for such care is specially trained midwives and nursing staff working in basic clinics accessible to the homes of the women.

An obstetrically trained doctor supervises them from the base hospital.

Strict criteria for referral of patients to the base hospital must be laid down and adhered to (see Suggested further reading).

High-risk patients may require immediate transfer to the hospital; emergency transport is therefore absolutely vital.

SUGGESTED FURTHER READING

Philpott R H (ed) 1982 Obstetric problems in the developing world. Clinics in obstetrics and gynaecology. Saunders, London, Vol 9, No. 3

SECTION TWO

Gynaecology

History and examination

SAMPLE CASE HISTORY

Name   Age   Unit number   Marital status

Patient's complaints

Past obstetric history

Parity

Details of any antenatal, intrapartum or postpartum problem

Date of last delivery

Past medical and surgical history

Social history: e.g. cigarettes smoked, alcohol intake

Relevant family history

Menstrual history

$$\text{Menstrual cycle (K)} = \frac{\text{length (days)}}{\text{interval (days)}}$$

Regular or irregular?   Blood loss — normal or abnormal (clots, pads/period)

LMP   Menarche

Contraceptive history: type(s) and for how long

Sexual history: dyspareunia — superficial or deep; constant or intermittent

GYNAECOLOGICAL SYMPTOMS

1. *Dysmenorrhoea*
   Always had it or developed (for how long?)
   Site
   Relationship to menses and duration
   Degree of incapacitation caused
   Relieved by what?
2. *Excessive bleeding* — use descriptive terms, e.g. heavy, irregular menses, rather than Latin or Greek terms, e.g. epimenorrhagia
3. *Inappropriate bleeding*:
   Intermenstrual
   Post-coital
   Post-menopausal

Enquire about use of hormones locally or systemically.

4. *Vaginal discharge* — colour, amount, duration, itching or irritant
5. *Urinary problems*
   Frequency or nocturia
   Dysuria
   Stress incontinence, urgency of micturition
6. *Pain or discomfort* (other than dysmenorrhoea)
   Site, duration, radiation and nature of pain
   Relationship to menses; other precipitating factors e.g. sharp pain in an iliac fossa in mid-cycle suggests ovulation pain
   Dragging discomfort in vagina or lower abdomen suggests prolapse
7. *Other symptoms*
   Gastrointestinal
   Cardiovascular
   Respiratory, etc.
8. *Current medication*

EXAMINATION

General: as indicated by history and intended management.
Breast: as a routine.
Abdomen: inspection, palpation, percussion (auscultation).
Pelvic: in either the dorsal or left lateral position.

1. Speculum examination

Using Cusco bivalve speculum if the patient is in the dorsal position, Sims' speculum for the left lateral position — this is particularly useful for assessing the extent of any utero-vaginal prolapse.

2. Bimanual examination

Uterus — size, shape, position, mobility, consistency, tenderness.
Adnexal regions — swellings? If so, note size, consistency, mobility, relationship to uterus. Tenderness?

3. Further tests

Cervical smear. Take cervical smear if the patient is (or has been) sexually active and has not had a smear for three years or more (p. 259)
Specimen of any discharge for microscopy
High vaginal or cervical swabs for bacteriology
Colposcopy if there is suspicion of cervical neoplasia
Suction aspiration of endometrium may allow diagnosis for

menstrual abnormalities without requiring admission for formal diagnostic curettage
Pelvic examination should *not* be carried out routinely in pre-pubertal children.
Summary: conclude by writing summary of history and examination.

Disorders of menstruation and associated problems

AMENORRHOEA

Definitions

1. No menstruation by the age of 14 years accompanied by failure to grow properly or develop secondary sexual characteristics
2. No menstruation by the age of 16 when growth and sexual development are normal

(These constitute primary amenorrhoea.)

3. The absence of menses for six months (or greater than three times the previous cycle intervals) in a woman who has menstruated before

(This is secondary amenorrhoea. When diagnoses are being considered, these 'primary' and 'secondary' categories must not be adhered to too rigidly.)

Causes

If the amenorrhoea is not physiological (pre-pubertal, pregnancy, post-menopausal) it may be due to:

1. Disorders of outflow tract and/or uterus
2. Disorders of ovary
3. Disorders of anterior pituitary
4. Disorders of hypothalamus

Disorder of outflow tract and/or uterus

1. Cryptomenorrhoea

Vaginal atresia or an imperforate hymen prevents menstrual loss from escaping.

Features. Primary amenorrhoea in a teenage girl with normal sexual development complaining of:

(i) Intermittent abdominal pain
(ii) Possible difficulty with micturition
(iii) Palpable lower abdominal swelling
(iv) Bulging, bluish membrane at lower end of vagina

Management: incise membrane under aseptic conditions.

2. Absence or hypoplasia of vagina
Features. Growth, development and ovarian function are usually normal. The uterus is usually absent if only the lower third of the vagina has developed but may be normal or rudimentary.
Renal anomalies (in 30%) or skeletal defects (in 10%) may be present also.

Management: a functional vagina can be created by surgery or by dilators.

3. Testicular feminisation
The phenotype is female but the genotype is XY, and testes are present. It is inherited by an X-linked recessive gene resulting in absence of cytosol androgen receptors.

Features:
(i) Growth and development are normal (may be taller than average and eunochoid)
(ii) Breasts are large but with sparse glandular tissue, nipples and pale areolae
(iii) Inguinal herniae occur in 50% of cases
(iv) Little or no axillary and pubic hair
(v) Labia minora are underdeveloped
(vi) The vagina is blind ending, the uterus absent and the fallopian tubes rudimentary
(vii) The testes are in the abdomen or inguinal canals
(viii) Normal levels of testosterone are produced but there is no response to androgens (endogenous or exogenous)
(ix) There is no spermatogenesis
(x) There is a high risk of testicular neoplasia (50%) if the testes are not removed shortly after puberty

Consider the diagnosis in a female child:
(i) With inguinal herniae
(ii) With primary amenorrhoea and absent uterus
(iii) When body hair is absent

Management: these patients should be treated as female. The gonads should be removed *after* puberty and oestrogen replacement therapy started.
Rare cases of incomplete testicular feminisation do occur. They have a variable degree of masculinisation.

4. Asherman's syndrome
Secondary amenorrhoea following destruction of the endometrium by overzealous curettage. Multiple synechiae show up on hysterography.
Management: break down intrauterine adhesions through a hysteroscope and insert an IUCD to deter reformation.

5. Infection
For example: tuberculosis and uterine schistosomiasis.

Disorders of the ovary

1. Chromosomal abnormalities
Turner's syndrome (45X) — gonadal dysgenesis.
Features:
(i) Amenorrhoea (primary but rarely secondary)
(ii) Short stature } most constant features
(iii) Failure of secondary sexual development
(iv) Webbing of the neck
(v) Increasing carrying angle
(vi) Shield chest
(vii) Coarctation of aorta } less common
(viii) Renal collecting system defects
Streak ovaries are present; gonadotrophins are high and oestrogens low.

A mosaic chromosome pattern (e.g. XX/XO) will lead to various degrees of gonadal dysgenesis, secondary amenorrhoea and premature menopause.

If a Y chromosome is present in the genotype the risk of gonadal malignancy makes gonadectomy advisable.

Management: short stature may be increased if the diagnosis is made early by use of oxandrolone and/or growth hormone *before* commencing oestrogen replacement therapy.

2. Failure of gonadal development — gonadal agenesis (see p. 234)

3. Resistant ovary syndrome
A rare condition in which FSH is elevated despite normal ovarian development and potential. It may resolve spontaneously — otherwise no treatment is possible except oestrogen therapy for any hot flushes.

4. Premature menopause
Ovarian failure before the age of 40 years occurs in 1% of women and may be due to:
(i) Auto-immune disease (associated with Addison's disease?)
(ii) Viral infection (e.g. mumps)
(iii) Cytotoxic drugs
(iv) Post-radiotherapy (most frequently for Hodgkin's disease)

Disorders of the pituitary

1. Pituitary tumours causing hyperprolactinaemia
About 40% of women with hyperprolactinaemia will have a

pituitary adenoma. Pituitary fossa X-rays must be taken in all cases of amenorrhoea. If coned views suggest any abnormality such as:

(i) Erosion of the clinoid processes
(ii) Enlargement of the fossa
(iii) Double flooring of the fossa

CT or MRI scanning and assessment of the visual fields are necessary.

Management: the dopamine agonist, bromocriptine, will suppress prolactin secretion, correct oestrogen deficiency, permit ovulation and reduce the size of most prolactinomas. The dosage should be increased slowly over several weeks to minimise side-effects (e.g. postural hypotension). In many centres surgical removal of tumours is now confined to those patients with extrasellar manifestations (e.g. pressure on the optic chiasma) or those who do not respond to or cannot tolerate bromocriptine.

An abnormal pituitary fossa may not be caused by a pituitary tumour but can be due to the *empty sella syndrome*. In this there is a congenital incompleteness of the diaphragma sellae and the subarachnoid space extends into the fossa. It is a benign condition.

2. Other causes of hyperprolactinaemia

A wide variety of drugs can cause it. Among the commonest are: phenothiazines, methyl-dopa, metoclopramide, antihistamines, oestrogen and morphine. It is also associated with hypothyroidism (with high TSH) and chronic renal failure.

In many patients no cause can be found.

3. Sheehan's syndrome

Necrosis of the anterior pituitary following severe postpartum haemorrhage. It is now very rare.

Disorders of the hypothalamus

The most common reason for hypogonadotrophic secondary amenorrhoea and often associated with weight loss, excessive exercise or stress. Diagnosed by exclusion of pituitary lesions.

Ovulation induction is not indicated unless the patient wishes to become pregnant. If a progestogen challenge test (e.g. medroxyprogesterone acetate 5 mg daily for 5 days) is negative, there is a significant risk of osteoporosis, and hormone replacement therapy should be given.

Weight loss-associated amenorrhoea

A loss of more than 10 kg is frequently associated with amenorrhoea. It usually occurs in young women (frequently teenagers); they become obsessed with their body image and starve themselves. Anorexia nervosa is a misnomer because there is no loss of appetite.

Oestrogen levels can be profoundly suppressed. Hypothalamo-pituitary-ovarian function is usually restored when the lost weight is regained but occasionally may take many months for normal cyclical activity to return and for amenorrhoea to resolve. Ovulation induction may be required but should be given only when weight >45 kg to avoid pregnancy risks (e.g. pre-term delivery).

Kallman's syndrome

A rare cause of hypogonadotrophic hypogonadism in which anosmia is associated with primary amenorrhoea. The underlying cause is an absence of LHRH.

Management: treatment with ethinyl oestradiol will induce normal secondary sexual development but the initial dosage should be $<7\ \mu g$/day to prevent premature epiphyseal fusion of long bones. Pulsatile LHRH therapy is a specific and reliable treatment for later ovulation induction.

Post-pill amenorrhoea

There is no evidence that the oestrogen/progestogen contraceptive pill predisposes to amenorrhoea once pill-taking ceases. An irregular menstrual cycle frequently precedes pill-taking. An assumption that amenorrhoea is merely an after-effect of pill-taking means that hyperprolactinaemia will be missed in one case from five and premature ovarian failure in one case from ten.

Once other underlying causes are excluded this type of amenorrhoea responds well to ovulation induction with clomiphene if pregnancy is desired.

Tumours

Rare causes include craniopharyngioma, or a mixed lesion producing acromegaly or Cushing's syndrome.

Basic investigation of amenorrhoea

1. Check serum prolactin level and thyroid function
2. If a chromosomal anomaly is likely on clinical grounds (e.g. short stature) check the karyotype
3. Progestogen challenge test (see above) to check endogenous oestrogen levels. The occurrence of withdrawal bleeding shows that the endometrium is reactive and the outflow tract patent

If the prolactin level is normal, and there is no galactorrhoea, further investigation for a pituitary tumour is unnecessary. Galactorrhoea requires evaluation of the pituitary regardless of prolactin levels or menstrual pattern.

If the prolactin level is significantly elevated a pituitary tumour must be excluded radiologically. Visual field assessment is necessary only if the X-rays are abnormal. If bleeding does not follow progestogen challenge measure FSH and LH. If they are in the normal range the diagnosis is pituitary inactivity or failure.

A low LH (<5 i.u./ml) suggests hypogonadotrophic hypogonadism. A high FSH (>40 i.u./ml) on successive readings indicates ovarian failure. If the woman is under 35 years of age check her karyotype. (The presence of a Y chromosome suggests that the risk of gonadal malignancy is high.)

4. Ultrasonic assessment of the uterus and ovaries (using a vaginal transducer if possible) can be useful to investigate and monitor treatment of these women

OLIGOMENORRHOEA

Definition

The occurrence of menses on only five or fewer occasions per year. Its causes are the same as those for secondary amenorrhoea, and if investigation is needed it should follow the same plan.

POLYCYSTIC OVARY DISEASE (PCOD)

A clinical syndrome of infertility, menstrual problems, hirsutism and obesity found to be associated with enlarged polycystic ovaries by Stein and Leventhal in 1935. It is not a single entity but rather a spectrum of disease.

High-resolution ultrasound will show the morphological feature of polycystic ovaries (multiple peripheral follicles <8 mm diameter and prominent echo-dense stroma) in up to 80% of anovulatory women.

Clinical features (in order of frequency)

1. Infertility
2. Hirsutism
3. Oligo-amenorrhoea
4. Obesity
5. Dysfunctional uterine bleeding
6. Virilisation
7. Family history of maturity onset diabetes

Despite the clinical evidence of excessive production of androgen there are no signs of oestrogen lack — the vaginal epithelium is healthy and the breasts are well developed.

Pathology

The ovaries are usually enlarged and show:

1. Numerous small cystic follicles (usually 5–6 mm in diameter but sometimes larger)
2. Thickened white ovarian capsule
3. Theca cell hyperplasia
4. Granulosa cell atresia

Endocrine abnormalities

1. Serum LH levels are increased, with FSH normal
2. An elevated free testosterone level is the commonest feature in PCOD (over 90% of cases)
3. Oestrogen levels are chronically high due to increased peripheral conversion
4. Sex hormone-binding globulin (SHBG) production is inhibited. This results in an increase in unbound (and therefore active androgen and oestradiol levels)
5. Peripheral insulin resistance commonly results in hyperinsulinaemia.

Pathogenesis

There is no general agreement about the exact mechanisms by which PCOD develops or continues:

1. Insulin resistance seems the most likely primary defect and may be inherited or acquired due to insulin receptor antibodies. A small proportion may be due to primary abnormalities of adrenal androgen production (e.g. 21-hydroxylase deficiency)
2. The resulting hyperinsulinaemia leads to amplification of the stroma-trophic effect of LH on the ovary, a small effect at the pituitary level increasing the production of LH, and a direct hepatic action which reduces SHBG production
3. The enhanced LH activity leads to an imbalance in ovarian steroidogenesis, with increased production of androgen (predominantly androstenedione and testosterone) by theca cells
4. Conversion of androgen to oestrogen within the follicle by granulosa cells is greatly reduced because of a *relative* deficiency of FSH and the excess enters the circulation
5. Aromatisation of the androgen surplus occurs peripherally in adipose tissue independently of FSH. This leads to a relatively constant oestrogen production with a larger than usual proportion of oestrone
6. Acyclic formation of oestrogen, particularly when unopposed by progesterone, results in abnormal feedback on the pituitary. FSH is suppressed and LH secretion promoted
7. The altered gonadotrophin profile distorts ovarian steroidogenesis further by accentuating theca cell hyperfunction and suppressing granulosa cell aromatase activity

The extent of which hirsutism occurs depends on the conversion of androgens to the active dihydrotestosterone by 5-alpha reductase

Oligo-amenorrhoea may occur, but otherwise the unopposed action of oestrogen leads to dysfunctional bleeding.

Management

This will depend on the primary problems.

1. If the woman is obese, loss of weight may be all that is necessary
2. Cycle control can be achieved by a low-dose combined oral contraceptive pill if she does not wish to conceive
3. Ovulation can usually be induced with clomiphene or tamoxifen but some women do not respond
4. Glucocorticoids are best reserved for the treatment of anovulation accompanied by adrenal hyperplasia
5. Treatment with HMG or pulsatile LHRH have been disappointing, but HMG following pituitary suppression with an LHRH analogue may be more successful
6. Low-dose FSH given subcutaneously by infusion pump may allow follicular maturation and, therefore, ovulation
7. Laparoscopic wedge resection of the ovaries or ovarian diathermy should be reserved for cases which have not responded to drug treatment or in which the size of the ovaries is causing symptoms. The way in which the wedge resection restores ovulation is not clear
8. Hirsutism is discussed below
9. Dysfunctional bleeding will usually respond to the combined oestrogen–progestogen pill or a progestogen only. This treatment will also reduce the increased risk of endometrial carcinoma occurring in these women due to prolonged unopposed oestrogen action

HIRSUTISM

Definition

Excessive and inappropriate growth of facial and body hair usually with a male pattern of distribution.

Causes

The most important causes are:

1. Endocrine — PCOD; adrenal hyperplasia/Cushing's syndrome; hypothyroidism; acromegaly
2. Androgen-secreting tumours of adrenal or ovary
3. Drugs — phenytoin, diazoxide, danazol, corticosteroids
4. Idiopathic

Investigation

1. Check serum testosterone — if <5 nmol/l no further investigation is required. If >5 nmol/l repeat and check

urinary steroids (cortisol and androgen metabolites in 24-hour sample)
2. Check serum LH, FSH and testosterone in early follicular phase. An elevated LH concentration and mildly elevated testosterone suggests PCOD
3. Pelvic ultrasound may demonstrate polycystic ovaries
4. Check thyroid function
5. Measure serum 17-hydroxyprogesterone if congenital adrenal hyperplasia is suspected. If levels are high consider ACTH simulation and dexamethasone suppression tests
6. If urinary cortisol is elevated investigate for Cushing's syndrome
7. If an adrenal tumour is suspected carry out CT or MRI scans and consider direct catheterisation of adrenal veins or surgical exploration

Treatment
This will depend on the cause. Sympathetic handling and reassurance are necessary at all times.
1. *Polycystic ovary disease* — induce ovulation if infertility is also a problem
   Otherwise, give a combined oestrogen/progestogen pill to suppress androgen production.
   Response to treatment is slow at best. It may be 6 months to a year before any reduction in hirsutes is seen. Cyproterone acetate is an anti-androgen with progestogenic activity. It will reduce hirsutes markedly in some but not all patients. Pregnancy must be avoided during its use. It is therefore best used cyclically (days 5–15) in combination with ethinyl oestradiol (days 5–26) which not only helps to inhibit ovulation but also increases SHBG concentrations. This lowers the levels of free androgens
2. *Adrenal hyperplasia*. This is the only situation in which corticosteroid treatment is clearly indicated
3. *Androgen-producing tumours* — remove after localisation
4. *Idiopathic hirsutism* — this may be due to end-organ hypersensitivity. There may be some response to the oestrogen/progestogen pill or cyproterone acetate and electrolysis is useful cosmetically

EXCESSIVE MENSTRUAL LOSS

Normal menstruation is defined as that occurring every 21–35 days, lasting 2–7 days and resulting in the loss of between 35 and 40 ml of blood.

Excessive loss can be due to menses which are too long, too frequent, too heavy, and/or too irregular.

Objective measurement of loss is not routinely practicable.

Causes

1. Physiological

Menorrhagia (regular, heavy menses) is a subjective complaint which may not be confirmed if blood loss were to be measured in all cases.

2. Dysfunctional uterine bleeding (60% of cases)

Abnormal bleeding from the uterus not due to organic disease. It can occur during:

(i) Anovulatory cycles

Features:

Usually a prolonged cycle ends in heavy, persistent vaginal bleeding but the menstrual pattern and loss can be very variable. It is commonest at the extremes of menstrual life. It can occur as part of the polycystic ovary syndrome. The older women who develop it are often obese (see below) and it is commoner when carbohydrate intolerance (e.g. maturity onset diabetes) is present

Pathogenesis

Near the menarche it is due to the failure to establish normal ovulatory cycles. It occurs even more commonly perimenopausally as ovulation begins to fail. Obesity leads to peripheral conversion of androgen to oestrogen (see polycystic ovary syndrome). It may be associated with other endocrine disorders, e.g. hypothyroidism, adrenal hyperplasia, acromegaly.

Pathology

The proliferative effects of oestrogen is unopposed by progesterone. The hyperplastic endometrium is shed when the ovarian follicle begins to degenerate or the endometrium outgrows its blood supply. In its most clearly defined form there is cystic glandular hyperplasia of the endometrium and the clinical result is known as metropathia haemorrhagica.

(ii) Ovulatory cycles

This problem is still not fully understood but is related to local disorders of prostaglandins and their receptors in the endometrium.

Features:

Heavy regular menses in the 35- to 45-year-old woman, often accompanied by lower abdominal discomfort, dysmenorrhoea and dyspareunia. The uterus is slightly enlarged and can be markedly tender to palpation.

Pathology

The endometrium is normal.

3. *Other gynaecological causes (35% of cases)*
 (i) Endometriosis — see p. 183
 (ii) Chronic pelvic inflammatory disease — see p. 218
 (iii) Uterine or ovarian tumours

Uterine:
- Benign — submucous leiomyomas (fibroids) (see p. 270) adenomatous polyps
  Rare tumours e.g. haemangioma, fibromas
- Malignant — carcinoma of the endometrium (see p. 273) may develop in cases of pre-existing endometrial hyperplasia

Ovarian: Theca cell and granulosa cell tumours often produce oestrogen (see p. 280)

 (iv) Intrauterine device (IUDs). The menstrual loss doubles in up to 50% of IUD users

4. *Endocrine and haematological causes* (<5% of case)
 (i) Thyroid disorders
 (ii) von Willebrand's disease and idiopathic thrombocytopenia (or rarely leukaemia) may present with menstrual disorders.
 Women on long-term anticoagulant therapy may have menorrhagia
Psychological factors can play an important part.
 (i) Post-sterilisation. If menstrual loss increases after sterilisation it may be because the woman has been on the C.O.C. pill and is therefore unaccustomed to normal menses.

MANAGEMENT OF EXCESSIVE MENSTRUAL LOSS

Investigation

A comprehensive history and examination is vital. A menstrual diary collected over several months can be helpful. Take blood for full blood count and film and check thyroid function and glucose tolerance as necessary.

Endometrial sampling should be carried out in women of 35 years of age or over. It is rarely necessary (or useful) in younger women. It can be frequently carried out as an outpatient procedure. *Note*: it is a diagnostic procedure which is virtually never therapeutic in even the short term.

Management

1. Specific organic disorders must be treated appropriately
2. The obese woman must be strongly advised to lose weight
3. Anovulatory cycles will usually respond to progestogen therapy from day 15 (or earlier) to 25 of the cycle. Young women can be given the combined oestrogen/progestogen pill

Dysfunctional bleeding associated with ovulatory cycles is much more difficult to manage in the long term. Among the suggested medical therapies are:

(i) Progestogen therapy is of no value and has side-effects (nausea, breast tenderness, water retention)
(ii) Prostaglandin synthetase inhibitors (e.g. mefenamic and flufenamic acids or naproxen sodium) will often reduce menstrual loss but the benefit gradually decreases over several cycles. Side-effects include headache, nausea and diarrhoea
(iii) *Antifibrinolytic therapy* (e.g. tranexamic acid) taken during menstruation may reduce the loss
(iv) *Ethamsylate* can reduce loss by reducing capillary fragility and inhibiting PG synthesis
(v) *Danazol* reduces loss but has many androgenic and other unwanted effects in over 75% of women who take it (see p. 218)

Conclusion: medical management is often unsuccessful.
Among the surgical remedies are:

(i) Endometrial ablation by Nd-YAG laser, cryosurgery, or electromagnetic radiation
(ii) Endometrial resection under hysteroscopic control

These have not yet been properly evaluated

(iii) Hysterectomy — there is no need to remove healthy ovaries as a matter of routine in older women

Endometrial hyperplasia
If the glands and stroma increase together and there are no atypical cells the risk of developing malignancy is under 2%. If hysterectomy is not carried out initially such women should be kept under observation by annual outpatient endometrial sampling. If the hyperplasia is atypical with abnormal cells in irregular glands the risk of endometrial adenocarcinoma is increased and hysterectomy is indicated.

DYSMENORRHOEA AND THE PREMENSTRUAL SYNDROME

Primary dysmenorrhoea

Definition
Painful periods for which no organic or psychological cause can be found.

Features:
It usually occurs in teenage girls. The pain is colicky and usually begins shortly after or at the onset of menses. It tends to last for only 24 to 48 hours. There is often an exacerbating

psychological element. There may be an increased production of prostaglandins. It occurs only in ovulatory cycles

Management

1. Exclude organic causes by history and examination
2. Suppression of ovulation using the combined oestrogen/progestogen pill may be helpful, or progestogens alone in the second half of the cycle
3. Symptomatic relief can often be obtained by prostaglandin synthetase inhibitors such as mefenamic and flufenamic acids or naproxen sodium
4. Procedures such as forced dilatation of the cervix or pre-sacral neurectomy are never indicated

Secondary dysmenorrhoea

Definition

Painful periods for which an organic or psychosexual cause can be demonstrated.

Features:

It usually commences in adult life. It begins several days before the menses and gradually increases in severity as menses approach. The commonest associations are with pelvic inflammatory disease, endometriosis, fibroids or psychosexual problems.

Management

1. Laparoscopy can be helpful in ascertaining the cause
2. The mainstay of treatment is to deal with the underlying cause

Premenstrual syndrome

A symptom complex of unknown aetiology occurring in the week before menstruation. The symptoms are an exaggerated form of those experienced by many women premenstrually.

Features:

Most frequent around the age of 35 years. Tension, irritability and depression can be marked. 'Fluid retention' causes a bloated feeling in the abdomen, breast tenderness and swollen clumsy fingers. There is an increased susceptibility to accidents, criminal acts and suicide among women during the premenstrual phase.

Management

1. Treatment is empirical because the cause is unknown
2. Sympathetic handling and understanding are of paramount importance

3. Progestogen therapy from mid-cycle may be of value
4. Pyridoxine (100 mg daily) may also provide some relief
5. Diuretics can reduce the fluid retention
6. LHRH agonists plus oestrogen may be useful for short-term treatment of severe cases
7. Hysterectomy and bilateral salpingo-oophorectomy may be necessary for a small group of women who are particularly severely affected

ENDOMETRIOSIS

Definition

The presence of endometrial tissue in sites other than the uterine cavity.

In internal endometriosis (adenomyosis) the ectopic endometrium is confined to the myometrium. External endometriosis, with deposits occurring in a variety of ectopic sites, is more common but is seldom found together with adenomyosis. This argues for different aetiological factors.

External endometriosis

Features:

It usually manifests itself between the ages of 30 and 40 years. Between 50 and 70% of the women will be nulliparous and most of the remainder of low parity. It is mostly confined to Caucasian women and is more prevalent in the higher socio-economic groups. The predominant symptoms are:

1. Heavy, often irregular menses
2. Secondary dysmenorrhoea
3. Dyspareunia
4. Pelvic pain between menses
5. Subfertility

There may also be symptoms relating to organs contiguous with the uterus.

Pathogenesis

There are several theories for its development:

1. Metaplasia — both epithelial and stromal cells of the endometrium have a common precursor in the coelomic epithelium and adjacent mesenchyme. This could account for all abdominal and pelvic endometriosis, and the rare cases in the rectovaginal septum, umbilicus and canal of Nuck
2. Retrograde menstruation and implantation of viable cells on, for example, the ovaries and peritoneum of the pouch of Douglas
3. Mechanical transplantation into scars at the time of surgery,

e.g. hysterectomy or hysterotomy. It very rarely follows Caesarean section
4. Venous or lymphatic 'metastasis'. This (or metaplasia) could account for the rare pulmonary endometriosis

It seems probable that all cases do not arise in the same way.

Pathology

The ectopic endometrium menstruates causing severe irritation, a sterile inflammatory reaction, and dense adhesions. The commonest sites are both ovaries, which may show merely surface deposits or contain 'chocolate' cysts (containing old menstrual blood) of various sizes. It is not clear whether the chocolate cysts arise by invagination of surface deposits or metaplasia of follicular or luteal cells. The next commonest sites are the pouch of Douglas and uterosacral ligaments. The pouch of Douglas may be obliterated but no matter how severe the surrounding adhesions the fallopian tubes remain open. The rectum may be involved which may cause rectal bleeding or painful defaecation at the time of the menses. It may be difficult to differentiate clinically from carcinoma. The secretions from the ectopic endometrium are luteolytic, which prevents establishment of the corpus luteum and therefore pregnancy leading to subfertility.

Diagnosis

It is often suspected after a careful history is taken. The presence of tender nodules on the uterosacral ligaments is also suggestive.

Laparoscopy is diagnostic but the significance of the occasional tiny deposits on e.g. the ovaries or pouch of Douglas is disputed.

For histological diagnosis both glandular and stromal tissue must be present.

Treatment

1. *Hormonal therapy* — this is the best approach to younger women wishing to achieve a pregnancy after treatment.
   (i) Continuous progestogen therapy for 6 to 9 months
   (ii) Danazol for 4 to 6 months. This drug interferes with gonadotrophin secretion, inhibits ovulation, and abolishes menses (or virtually so). It has androgenic side-effects and must be discontinued if signs of virilisation develop.

   Weight gain may occur due to mild anabolic affect and fluid retention. Muscle cramps are not uncommon. It does not usually affect libido.

   It must not be used in pregnancy and caution is

advised when liver, heart or renal problems are present. It potentiates the action of anticoagulants
2. Vaporisation of endometriotic deposit by CO_2 laser at laparoscopy (see Suggested further reading)
3. *Conservative surgery*. Small deposits can be diathermied or excised. Large chocolate cysts require excision
4. *Hysterectomy and bilateral salpingo-oophorectomy*. These must not be embarked on too lightly because the surgery can be very difficult. Prior treatment with danazol or LHRH agonists may be worthwhile in severe cases. Both ovaries must be removed or residual endometriosis will continue to give problems. Oestrogen implants should not be used at surgery for the same reason but, if menopausal symptoms become troublesome, oral hormone replacement therapy can be given

Adenomyosis
Islets of endometrial tissue, glands and stroma are found deep in the uterine wall which responds by hyperplasia of muscle and fibrous tissue.

Features:
It tends to occur in older, more multiparous women, in contrast to external endometriosis. The clinical presentation is:
1. Increasingly severe menorrhagia
2. Secondary dysmenorrhoea
3. Gradually enlarging tender uterus

Symptomatically it is difficult to differentiate from uterine fibroids or dysfunctional bleeding
The uterus may be diffusely thickened or there may be localised swellings closely resembling leiomyomas
It is virtually impossible to diagnose it definitely without first removing the uterus and obtaining a histology report on it

Treatment
Hysterectomy with conservation of ovaries (unless there are other indications for their removal).

Stromal endometriosis
This rare condition acts more like a neoplasm than do other forms of endometriosis.

Histologically, solid masses of cells resembling endometrial stroma are found in the endometrial wall, but other features of neoplasm are uncommon (e.g. mitoses are few and pleomorphism slight).

Features:
The peak incidence is between the ages of 35 and 50 years

It does not regress on removal of the ovaries
Metastases do occur, but rarely, and it has been thought to be a low-grade sarcoma; this seems likely
Clinically it may present with:

1. Menorrhagia or postmenopausal bleeding
2. Pelvic pain

It is usually diagnosed only after hysterectomy. The prognosis is usually good.

SUGGESTED FURTHER READING

Jacobs H S (ed) 1985 Reproductive endocrinology. Clinics in obstetrics and gynaecology. Saunders, London, Vol 12, No. 3
Schneider G T 1983 in Studd J. (ed) Progress in obstetrics and gynaecology. Churchill Livingstone, Edinburgh, p. 246, Vol 3
Speroff L, Glass R H, Kase N G 1989 Clinical gynaecologic endocrinology and infertility, 4th edn. Williams and Williams Co., Baltimore
Sutton C J G 1989 Laparoscopic surgery. Clinical Obstetrics and Gynaecology 3: 499–523
Tindall V R 1990 Jeffcoate's principles of gynaecology. 5th edn. Butterworths, London

Fertility and subfertility

FERTILITY IN THE FEMALE

The hypothalamus

Controls anterior pituitary function by substances secreted by cells within it and transported to the pituitary *via* the portal circulation

1. A single decapeptide neurotransmitter controls FSH and LH-gonadotrophin-releasing hormone (GnRH). Its half-life is only a few minutes, and a continuous but pulsatile release occurs. Release is controlled by:
   (i) A long feedback loop due to circulating target gland hormones
   (ii) A short feedback loop due to the effect of gonadotrophins on the hypothalamus
   (iii) An ultrashort feedback by which it inhibits its own synthesis
   (iv) A series of neurotransmitters such as serotonin, melatonin, noradrenaline and dopamine (see below)

The hypothalamus exerts a tonic negative control on prolactin through the major *prolactin inhibitory factor*, dopamine.

The pituitary gland

It is influenced by the hypothalamus via:

1. *Tonic and cyclic centres for the secretion of GnRh*
   The tonic centre is responsible for basal levels of gonadotrophin. Oestradiol has a negative feedback effect on it and it is also dopamine-dependent. It is situated in the medial basal hypothalamus.
   The cyclic centre is responsive to positive feedback by oestradiol and produces the mid-cycle surge of gonadotrophins. It lies in the pre-optic area in the anterior part of the hypothalamus
2. *The posterior pituitary pathway*
   Cells in the supraoptic and paraventricular nuclei secrete vasopressin, oxytocin and neurophysin. They are transported

along the pituitary stalk to the posterior pituitary where they are stored in axonal terminals. They also pass into the CSF and then to the portal system of the anterior pituitary. Oxytocin is involved in gonadotrophin secretion

Gonadotrophin release
There are two pools, one released immediately it is synthesised and the other held in reserve. The rate of storage exceeds release, which makes the mid-cycle surge possible. (This is also the time when sensitivity to GnRh is greatest.) Oestradiol inhibits immediate release and increases storage. The effect is overcome by the positive feedback action of oestradiol on the cyclic centre. Low levels of progesterone increase release and storage after oestrogen priming. High levels of progesterone increase GnRH pulse frequency. The release of LH is pulsatile, and of FSH non-pulsatile.

Regulation of the menstrual cycle

Recruitment of follicles (days 2–6)
Initiation of follicular growth is independent of gonadotrophin stimulation. Follicles grow during infancy, ovulation, periods of anovulation, pregnancy and the menopause until the numbers are exhausted. For the vast majority of follicles growth is limited and atresia inevitable. As FSH levels increase, a group of follicles begins to grow further but the mechanism by which these follicles is chosen is unknown. The period of initial growth ends as oestrogen levels rise seven to eight days before the pre-ovulatory LH surge.

Selection of follicles (days 7–10)
FSH stimulates follicular growth but also facilitates steroidogenesis by increasing the activity or number of LH receptors. Changes in hormonal levels are regulated by feedback mechanisms:
1. Oestradiol inhibits FSH (negative feedback)
2. Low levels of oestradiol inhibit LH
3. High levels of oestradiol stimulate LH (positive feedback) and FSH

Dominant follicle selection (days 10–14)
Oestrogens rise slowly, the rapidly, to peak just before ovulation. FSH falls due to negative feedback. LH increases steadily to its mid-cycle surge. The follicle destined to ovulate protects itself by its own hormone production. Ovarian stromal cell production of androgens (androstenedione and testosterone) increases — enhancing the atresia of non-ovulatory follicles and stimulating libido.

Ovulation
The rapid rise in oestrogen triggers an LH and FSH surge. The LH surge triggers resumption of meiosis by the oocyte. Degeneration of the collagen in the follicular wall allows it to rupture. Expulsion of the oocyte is brought about by prostaglandins induced by LH, and hormones such as noradrenaline and relaxin.

Luteal phase
1. Days 1–3 post-ovulation: granulosa cells increase in size, accumulate lutein (a yellow pigment) and secrete progesterone
2. Days 8–9 post-ovulation: peak levels of progesterone and oestradiol are reached

(A plasma level of progesterone over 30 nmol/l (10 ng/ml) is good presumptive evidence of ovulation.)

3. Days 9–11 post-ovulation: the corpus luteum begins to decline unless pregnancy supervenes. Regression may be due to a local luteolytic effect or to oestradiol production by the CL. In pregnancy it is maintained by hCG until 6 to 8 weeks gestation
4. In the absence of pregnancy the time from the LH surge to the onset of menstrual flow is usually 14 days

FERTILITY IN THE MALE

The testes have two functions:
1. *Steroidogenesis* by the interstitial cells of Leydig between the seminiferous tubules
2. *Spermatogenesis,* which begins in the germinal epithelium of the tubules

The seminiferous tubules and interstitial cells are controlled by:
1. *GnRH and gonadotrophins*
2. *Positive and negative feedback signals*
   Testicular steroids (particularly oestrogen) inhibit GnRH
   Androgens diminish the LH-releasing effect of GnRH without affecting FSH
   Oestrogen potentiates FSH and LH secretion by GnRH
   Seminiferous tubules secrete *inhibin,* a non-steroid substance, which specifically inhibits FSH release
   The effects of androgens are:
   (i) Spermatogenesis
   (ii) Development of accessory glands
   (iii) Development of secondary sex characteristics
   (iv) Metabolic and psychic effects determining 'maleness'
   (v) Increasing sexual appetite
   (vi) Feedback on the hypothalamus and pituitary (see above)

Erection

Erection is due to tumescence of the penile cavernous bodies. It is mediated through the parasympathetic nervi erigentes (S2–4).

Ejaculation

Ejaculation is a reflex action involving a complex co-ordinated autonomic stimulation of the genital tract. It has two stages:

1. Contractions of the epididymis, vas deferens and seminal vesicle pump sperm from the epididymis and seminal fluid from the prostate and seminal vesicles into the posterior urethra. As the seminal fluid arrives in the prostatic urethra contraction of the internal urethral sphincter closes the bladder neck (this prevents retrograde ejaculation). The second stage is triggered
2. The semen is expelled due to relaxation of the external sphincter and rhythmic contractions of ischiocavernous, bulbo-cavernous and perineal muscles

Testicular function and age

Gonadal function in men is preserved well into old age and any decline is gradual.

Although FSH and LH levels remain normal, testosterone levels tend to fall, suggesting decreased sensitivity to gonadotrophin.

The so-called 'male climacteric' is more likely to be related to psychological, cardiovascular and neurological effects of ageing than to diminished production of androgens.

SUBFERTILITY

Definition: The involuntary failure to conceive within 12 months of commencing unprotected intercourse.

Primary subfertility — no previous pregnancy
Secondary subfertility — previous pregnancy (whatever the outcome)

Incidence of primary subfertility alone is at least 12% of married couples.

Causes (and approximate incidence)

1. Idiopathic	25%
2. Sperm defects or functional disorder	25%
3. Ovulation failure	20%
4. Tubal damage	15%
5. Endometriosis	5%
6. Coital failure	5%
7. Cervical mucus defect	3%
8. Azoospermia	2%

Aims of investigation

An explanation for the infertility

A prognosis
A basis for treatment

Principles of management
Deal with the infertile couple together. No one is 'at fault' or 'to blame'

Carry out investigations and treatments consistently in proper sequence.

Investigations

History — check:

Both partners	Past medical, surgical and family histories For sexually transmitted disease Coital history
Female	Previous pregnancies Menstrual history Galactorrhoea Hirsutism
Male	Mumps orchitis Occupation — excess heat, radiation, toxic chemicals, sedentary job?

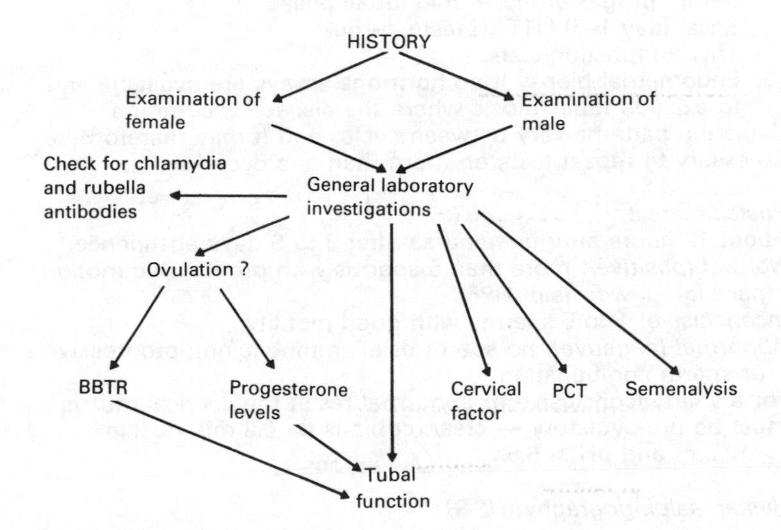

Examination

Female	Look for signs of endocrine or other systemic diseases, hirsutism and tumours and genital abnormalities. Carry out general examination. Perform postcoital test (PCT) and cervical score (see below)

Male — Look for signs of endocrine or other systemic diseases, lack of virilisation and genital abnormalities including testicular size, epididymal cysts and varicocoeles

Routine investigation in the female

General

Check for *Chlamydia* and Rubella antibody levels. If the latter is negative, immunise and advise against pregnancy for 3 months.

Investigation of ovulation

1. Basal body temperature recording (BBTR). A temperature rise in mid-cycle sustained for about 14 days suggests that ovulation may have taken place, but it is not an accurate index of progesterone levels. The following features may suggest, but are not diagnostic of, abnormal ovulation patterns: monophasic (perhaps an inability to take temperature), slow rise in temperature, short elevation of temperature
2. Hormone assays
   Serum prolactin
   Serum progesterone — mid-luteal phase
   Basal (day 1–5) LH/FSH/testosterone
   Thyroid function tests
3. Endometrial biopsy if no hormone assays are available and to exclude tuberculosis where the disease is common

Ovulation patterns vary between cycles and it may therefore be necessary to repeat tests on more than one occasion.

Postcoital test

About 12 hours after intercourse after 3 to 5 days abstinence.
Normal (positive): more than 5 sperms with progressive motion per high-power field (HPF).
Inconclusive: 1 to 5 sperms with good motility.
Abnormal (negative): no sperm *or* all immobile/non-progressive *or* sperm agglutination.
For a valid inconclusive or abnormal result the cervical mucus must be pre-ovulatory — clear, copious (> 0.3 ml), ductile (> 10 cm) and pH > 6.5.

Hysterosalpingography (HSG)

Indications

1. History/examination suggest tubal damage or if chlamydial antibody titres are elevated
2. Other investigations abnormal or infertility persists despite treatment
3. Previous surgery on uterus or tubes

Patient must avoid pregnancy in HSG cycle. General anaesthetic is seldom necessary. Buscopan i.v. can be given to counteract tubal spasm.

Routine investigation in the male

Semenalysis

Test after 3 days abstinence from intercourse. Three readings a month apart are necessary to confirm abnormality.

Normal values:

Volume	2 to 6 ml
Density	20 to 250 $\times 10^6$/ml
Motility	$>$ 50% with forward motion within 2 hours
Morphology	$>$ 50% normal sperm

Other features to be noted are:

- Viscosity
- Liquefaction
- Sperm clumping
- Presence of inflammatory cells

Anti-sperm antibodies can be tested for using the *mixed erythrocyte–spermatozoa antiglobulin reaction* (MAR test). Anti-Rh antibodies and semen are mixed with Rh-positive erythrocytes. If spermatozoa carry antisperm antibodies they are caught up in the agglutination reaction.

Further management in the female

Induction of ovulation

Defective ovulation can be due to:

1. Non-specific hypothalamo-pituitary dysfunction
2. Hyperprolactinaemia
3. Polycystic ovarian disease (see p. 175)
4. Other endocrine disorders

Amenorrhoeic women

If the patient is amenorrhoeic with normal prolactin and gonadotrophin levels carry out a progestogen challenge test.

If no withdrawal bleeding follows Provera 5 mg b.d. for 5 days, gonadotrophin or pulsatile GnRH therapy is likely to be necessary.

If withdrawal bleeding occurs therapy with oral fertility agents is indicated (see below).

Women having menstrual cycles (however irregular)

If progesterone level in the luteal phase are low prescribe clomiphene or tamoxifen (see below).

Check progesterone levels again in the second treatment cycle. If normal ovulation is still not occurring the dose of clomiphene or tamoxifen can be increased.

If there is still no ovulation check plasma oestrogen levels and/or follicular growth using ultrasound in the follicular phase.

A good rise in oestrogen or follicular growth without ovulation or failure of any oestrogen response or follicular growth suggests that gonadotrophin therapy is likely to be necessary.

If pregnancy does not occur within six treatment cycles despite good ovulation review other factors critically (but continue therapy).

Oral fertility agents

These compete with natural oestrogens by blocking receptors in target organs, including the pituitary, leading to increased FSH levels. Follicles develop and ovulation follows in 85% of well-oestrogenised women.

1. *Clomiphene*. The dose is 50 to 150 mg daily from days 2 to 6 or days 5 to 9 of the cycle. Side-effects are few: visual disturbances may occur
2. *Tamoxifen*. The dose is 10 to 40 mg twice daily for five days as above. Side-effects are few

The incidence of miscarriage and twins is slightly increased. There may be an increased incidence of abnormalities but only when the drug is taken inadvertently after conception.

Ovarian hyperstimulation is rare and resolves spontaneously.

Gonadotrophin therapy

This is indicated in women with hypogonadotrophic hypogonadism who are resistant to oral agents or pulsatile GnRH.

Occasional and casual use is dangerous because:

1. Ovarian sensitivity varies between cycles and patients
2. The difference in dose between normal ovulation and hyperstimulation is small
3. The rate of multiple conceptions and miscarriage is high unless control is meticulous

Human menopausal gonadotrophin (HMG) or purified FSH is used to develop the follicle.

Human chorionic gonadotrophin (HCG) induces ovulation. Treatment should be monitored by urinary or plasma oestrogen and ultrasound measurement of follicular growth (number and size).

Multiple pregnancy rate — between 12 and 45% depending on the degree of control. If good, 75% of the multiple pregnancies are twins. Anything higher is a failure of treatment.

Hyperstimulation

Mild in 6% of cases. Severe in 2% of cases.

Mild — excess oestrogen output with ovarian enlargement; no cysts; some abdominal pain. No treatment needed.

Moderate — detectable but not large ovarian cysts; abdominal pain, nausea, vomiting, diarrhoea. Admit for observation and symptomatic treatment.

Severe — large ovarian cysts, ascites (possibly hydrothorax) Severe abdominal pain and distension. Possible thrombo-embolism due to haemoconcentration.

Management: correct fluid and electrolyte imbalance (avoid diuretics). Intravenous colloid should be used for infusion rather than crystalloid. Screen for early evidence of DIC. Laparotomy only if cysts have ruptured or are bleeding.

Gonadotrophin releasing hormone (GnRH or LHRH)
Pulsatile subcutaneous (or intravenous) infusion of GnRH by miniaturised automatic infusion systems has been successful in clomiphene-resistant anovulation. Endocrine events in the normal cycle are mimicked and the multiple pregnancy rate is low.

Treatment is monitored using ultrasound measurement of follicular development. After ovulation the pulsatile infusion may be discontinued and luteal phase support may be given by a single injection of hCG. It is usually ineffective in women with PCOD (see p. 175).

Hyperprolactinaemia
The potential causes are discussed on p. 172

1. *Slight to moderate elevation* — repeat the estimation, and if it is still elevated carry out X-ray examination of the pituitary fossa.
2. *Marked elevation* — repeat the test but arrange skull X-ray forthwith. Check visual fields

If the skull X-ray is abnormal or prolactin levels are very high (>2500 μmol/l) arrange CT scan or tomography.

Evaluation of the cervical factor

PCT	*Action*
Normal	Cervix not implicated
No sperm	Sperm in vaginal pool? If no — psychosexual problem If yes — perform SIT/crossed penetration test
Sperm dead or clumped	Check for anti-sperm antibodies in wife. Perform SIT/crossed penetration test
	Endocervical swabs for routine organisms and *Neisseria*, *Mycoplasma* or *Chlamydia*

SIT = sperm invasion test.

Causes of abnormal SIT	*Treatment*
Endocervicitis	Antibiotics Cryocautery to cervix
Failure of cervix to respond to endogenous oestrogen	Ethinyl oestradiol 100 μg daily for 10 days from start of cycle and repeat PCT. A positive result is an indication for gonadotrophin therapy. If negative, consider assisted conception (p. 194)
Anti-sperm antibodies in semen or mucus	None of proven efficacy

Treatment (see p. 177)

Results of ovulation induction therapy
The cumulative conception rate after 2 years is 95% for amenorrhoeic women and 80% for those with oligomenorrhoea (when these are the sole disorders).

Tubal factors
HSG and laparoscopy are complementary investigations of tubal function.

Indications for laparoscopy
1. Abnormal HSG
2. History or examination suggest need for direct investigation, e.g. endometriosis
3. All other investigations normal or abnormal but corrected — in such cases unsuspected problems can be found in 30%

Peritubal adhesions — avascular adhesions can be divided at laparoscopy or laparotomy (salpingolysis). Treatment of vascular adhesions gives poor results.

Tubal blockage — surgery for mild/moderate damage, IVF if severe.

Salpingostomy — surgical opening of ostia. Conception rate no more than 20%.

Excision of block and re-anastomosis — conception rate 10 to 15%.

The incidence of ectopic pregnancies is increased in treated cases.

Concurrent hysteroscopy and salpingoscopy will exclude occult endometrial pathology and assess damage to the endosalpinx.

Further management in the male
Present understanding of infertility problems in the male is poor and treatment very disappointing.

Erectile impotence

May be due to:

(i) Vascular disease, e.g. secondary to smoking

(ii) Hyperprolactinaemia

Azoospermia

This may be due to:

1. *Ejaculatory failure*
   (i) Exclude retrograde ejaculation by examining urine postcoitally
   (ii) If psychogenic impotence is present refer for psychosexual counselling
   (iii) Consider neurological disorders — e.g. multiple sclerosis, diabetic neuropathy, urological factors and drug side-effects (e.g. antihypertensive therapy)
2. *Failure of spermatogenesis*
   Assess testicular size — more likely if volume <15 ml by orchidometer.
   Check FSH levels. Significant elevation is found in:
   (i) Klinefelter's syndrome (therefore check karyotype)
   (ii) Spermatogenic arrest
   (iii) Sertoli cell only syndrome
   (iv) Testicular atrophy
   There is no remedy for any of these problems.
3. *Obstruction*
   If testicular size and consistency and FSH are normal consider congenital or acquired block of the vasa by semen biochemistry (see below) and/or vasography
4. *Hypogonadotrophism*
   This is indicated by lack of virilisation, impotence and reduced testosterone level with normal or low FSH and LH levels. This is the only treatable cause of azoospermia. The regimen is HMG 1 to 3 ampoules daily for 110 days and HCG 5000 units weekly. Because spermatogenesis takes over 70 days treatment must be prolonged. Once spermatogenesis has been stimulated HCG alone will maintain sperm counts. Pulsed GnRH is an alternative but impractical for such prolonged use

Oligospermia

This is often accompanied by seminal plasma of high viscosity and/or low volume which fails to liquefy. Low sperm density and poor motility are related disorders.

Seminal biochemistry may indicate the source of the problem. Elevated FSH levels (>8 i.u./l) suggest irreversible sterility. Low levels of testosterone and high LH levels are frequently secondary to severe testicular damage which is irreversible.

Seminal biochemistry

Acid phosphatase, zinc	*Fructose*	*Carnitine*	*Possible site of defect*
Absent	Present	Present	Prostate
Present	Absent	Present	Seminal vesicles
Present	Present	Absent	Epididymis

Testicular biopsy is of little practical, diagnostic or therapeutic value.

Cytogenetic studies. Karyotype will reveal abnormalities in up to 6% of infertile males and 20% when azoospermia is present. No treatment is available apart from donor insemination (DI).

Therapy for oligospermia. There is no proven effective drug treatment. All claims for success using clomiphene or mesterolone must be compared with the spontaneous pregnancy rate in oligospermic men.

High ligation of a varicocoele improves semenalysis in 60% of cases but is of no proven benefit for conception.

Artificial insemination

1. Husband (AIH) — only when intercourse is impossible due to male impotence or anatomical defects but a normal ejaculate can be obtained
2. Donor insemination (DI) — the greatest care must be taken to:
   (i) Protect the identity of the donors
   (ii) Ascertain that both husband and wife are sure they wish this form of treatment

Inseminations are usually carried out twice in the peri-ovulatory phase. Prior investigation of female infertility is mandatory; checking for stress-induced ovulatory dysfunction during the initial 2–3 treatment cycles is advisable.

Assisted conception

In vitro fertilisation (IVF)

It is estimated that up to 20% of subfertile couples could benefit from IVF. It is most applicable amongst women with tubal blockage or damage, or those with unexplained subfertility. It is relatively inefficient for male subfertility and is entirely inappropriate for ovulatory disorders.

It is expensive and requires sophisticated laboratory facilities and highly skilled medical, nursing, scientific and technical personnel. If it is to be established within the NHS, regional centres should be set up operating under strict control.

Suggested guidelines for proceeding with assisted conception

1. Clear positive recommendation from GP

2. No more than one previous child
3. A continuing stable heterosexual relationship of at least 2 years' duration
4. Treatment is technically feasible with a good chance of success, e.g. not in women of 40 years of over?
5. Couples in good health such that both can be reasonably expected to bring up the child together
6. Appropriate domestic and social circumstances

These guidelines could, in fact, be applied to the whole problem of infertility.

Outline protocol for IVF

1. Multiple ovulation is induced with HMG after pituitary down-regulation with an LHR analogue to inhibit any endogenous LH rise. Alternatively, clomiphene and HMG may be given. Follicular maturation is monitored ultrasonically and by urinary or plasma oestrogen levels
2. Mature oocytes are recovered just before ovulation (following an injection of HCG) by laparoscopy. The aim is to collect at least four eggs. Transvaginal aspiration of follicles under ultrasound guidance is frequently used (under i.v. sedation)
3. Fertilisation of ovum by sperm occurs within 24 hours in a fluid culture medium at physiological temperature and atmospheric conditions. There is a 70% chance of each mature egg being fertilised
4. Embryos are transferred to the uterus through the cervical canal after 2 to 3 days (i.e. around the eight-cell stage)

Gamete intra-Fallopian transfer (GIFT)

GIFT is suitable for all women who are candidates for IVF except those with blocked or damaged Fallopian tubes. Oocytes are collected as above by laparoscopy or mini-laparotomy, mixed with 5×10^5 sperm in buffered medium and transferred into the fimbrial end of the tube.

GIFT is theoretically superior to IVF because fertilisation occurs in the normal site and implantation at the normal time (5–6 days) after ovulation (cf. IVF at 2 days). This is reflected in the greater number of pregnancies and births with GIFT than in IVF (see below). It too is expensive, and the conditions for setting it up should be as for IVF.

Intrauterine insemination (IUI)

IUI using husband's semen after superovulation of the woman can be useful in some cases. When used appropriately about 20% of the women will become pregnant and 15% will have a child.

Ovum donation followed by IVF
This can be used with the same considerations as for DI (p. 198) in women who:

Have had their ovaries removed
Have experienced premature menopause } Appropriate hormonal support is required
or Who carry a serious genetic defect

Results of IVF and GIFT
Transfer of a single embryo results in a pregnancy in less than 10% of cases. It is therefore usual to transfer three embryos, which gives a 25 to 30% chance of a single pregnancy, a 5% chance of twins, and a 1 to 2% chance of triplets.

The overall efficiency of the method (the 'take-home baby rate') is between 15 and 20% for each cycle. This probably does not differ significantly from conception rates in normal couples.

About 20% of women will have a child per cycle of IVF treatment compared with about 30% for GIFT.

SUGGESTED FURTHER READING

Behrman S J, Kistner R W, Patton G W (eds) 1988 Progress in infertility. 3rd edn. Little Brown & Co, Boston

Speroff L, Glass R H, Kase N G 1989 Clinical gynaecologic endocrinology and infertility. 4th edn. Williams and Wilkins, Baltimore

Contraception and sterilisation

Human fertility can be measured in several ways, e.g.:

General fertility rate — this is the number of births during a year per 1000 women of childbearing age.

Age-specific fertility rate — the number of births during a year occurring to women of a specified five-year age group per 1000 women of that age range.

Total fertility rate — the average size of a completed family.

Contraceptive effectiveness can also be measured. This is traditionally done by means of the Pearl index which expresses failures in terms of the numbers of pregnancies per 100 woman-years (w.y.) of exposure.

The more exact life-table method of assessment takes varying periods of contraceptive use into account and provides cumulative rates for either pregnancy or continuation of use of the contraceptive method per 100 users by the end of the stated period of time (e.g. the first year).

The use-effectiveness is the most important in practice because it takes into account the vagaries of human nature and other real-life situations.

STEROIDAL CONTRACEPTION

Steroidal contraception has, as its basis, synthetic oestrogens and progestogens.

Pharmacology

The oestrogen in most pills is now ethinyloestradiol. Much attention has been paid to the development of progestogens which bind more specifically to progesterone receptors and have less effect on sex hormone-binding globulin (SHBG) and high-density lipoprotein (HDL). They are thus less anti-oestrogenic and may reduce the risk of arterial disease. Such progestogens include desogestrel, gestodene and norgestimate. The effect of any one combined oral contraceptive (COC) will depend on the balance of the oestrogen and progestogen it contains. It appears possible to reduce the dose of ethinyloestradiol to 20 μg when used with desogestrol without loss of contraceptive effect.

Mode of action

1. Inhibition of ovulation due to negative feedback on the hypothalamo-pituitary-ovarian axis
2. Induction of changes in cervical mucus, endometrium, myometrium and Fallopian tubes which makes them hostile to sperm and unfavourable for ovum transplant and implantation

Types of steroidal contraceptives

1. *Combined oral contraceptives (COC)* are the most widely used:
   (i) Monophasic (fixed dose) pills. Oestrogen and progestogen are taken in constant doses for 21 days followed by an interval of 7 days
   (ii) Preparations containing phased doses of oestrogen and progestogen. Norethisterone- and norgestrel-containing pills are available in this form in the UK. The bio-availability of steroid varies up to 10 times in individual women, and the range of preparations available make it possible to 'titrate' the dose to the individual woman in order to find the lowest dose of both hormones that will provide good cycle control, and least side-effects.
2. *Continuous low-dose oral progestogens (POP)* have a good contraceptive effect provided they are taken regularly 3–4 hours before expected intercourse. Ovulation is only inhibited in 40% of women, and the anti-fertility effect on cervical mucus which wears off after 16–20 hours is important. Despite being less effective than the COC the failure rate can be as low as 0.9 per 100 w.y. in older women. Irregular menstruation is frequent but improves as use continues. Some patients develop amenorrhoea. POPs increase the risk of functional ovarian cysts (see p. 277).

   The incidence of ectopic pregnancies is still in dispute. The POP may produce a genuine increase because of its effect on the Fallopian tube, or it may be less effective in preventing ectopic pregnancies than intrauterine ones. Where possible the COC or injectable progestogen (which inhibits ovulation) should be used in those with a past history of ectopic pregnancy.

   Lactation is not inhibited by POP and there does not appear to be an effect on blood pressure. They are particularly suitable for lactating women, diabetics, those with contra-indications or intolerance to oestrogen, and possibly, those with a past history of venous thrombosis. They deserve to be more widely used.

3. *Injectable steroids* given as intramuscular injections of e.g. medroxyprogesterone acetate (Depo-Provera) 150 mg every 3 months or norethisterone oenanthate 200 mg every 8 weeks. They are highly effective. Effects on glucose tolerance and plasma lipids are markedly less than those caused by COC. Occasionally there is some weight gain. There appears to be no effect on blood pressure or blood coagulability. Menstruation tends to be irregular and may be prolonged. Heavy vaginal bleeding is rare.

   Amenorrhoea will supervene in about a third of users within 1 year. Despite more than 10 million users over 15 years no increased risk of carcinoma of breast, endometrium or cervix have been noted. Menstrual cycles and fertility return to normal within 6 months of the last injection.

   If used during lactation the quality and quantity of milk is improved. Only a tiny quantity of steroid is ingested by the infant and as yet no adverse effects have been noted.

   Precautions must be taken to ensure that the injection is not given to an already pregnant woman.

4. *Implants and vaginal rings.* Much work is being done on alternate delivery systems which avoid the 'first-pass' effect of the oral route. Progestogen only and combined hormone releasing rings are at an advanced stage of development, as are progestogen releasing implants.

5. *Postcoital preparations.* The most successful of these is ethinyloestradiol 100 μg and levonorgestrel 500 μg taken within 72 hours of unprotected intercourse and repeated 12 hours later.

   Nausea and vomiting are common. It is not recommended as a routine method but is an invaluable emergency method, including following rape.

Metabolic changes

Glucose tolerance is reduced particularly by the use of the combined pill but also to a much lesser extent by the progestogen-only pill.

If used in women with established diabetes, therapy may well require modification, and overt disease may be induced in women with latent diabetes.

Women on the combined pill sometimes complain of weight gain but double-blind studies fail to demonstrate this clearly.

There is conflicting evidence about the effect of the combined pill on lactation. It is, however, best to use progestogen-only (or other) contraception while breast-feeding is continuing.

Beneficial non-contraceptive side-effects of COC
Less menorrhagia and dysmenorrhoea
Less anaemia
Carcinoma of endometrium and ovary reduced by at least 50%; this effect may increase with duration of use, and continues after stopping
Reduced risk of pelvic inflammatory disease
Reduced benign breast disease
Reduced ovarian cysts
Reduced ectopic pregnancy
Possible protective effect against fibroids, rheumatoid arthritis and duodenal ulcer

Adverse effects of COC

1. *Metabolic effects*
   (i) *Carbohydrate metabolism* is affected by contraceptive steroids, but modern low-oestrogen and progestogen preparations produce minor effects on insulin secretion and little or no change in glucose tolerance. Significant glucose intolerance occasionally occurs in susceptible individuals and insulin-dependent diabetics may need to increase their dose
   (ii) *Lipid metabolism*. High lipid concentrations are associated with an increased risk of cardiovascular disease, and the ratios of LDL and total cholesterol to HDL cholesterol are important indicators of risk. The effect of oestrogen/progestogen combinations depends on the type of progestogen and the relative doses. The aim of modern pills is to have a near-neutral effect, but long-term epidemiological studies are needed to confirm that these pills have lower risks
   (iii) *Haemostatic factors*. Changes in the coagulation system produced by COC are complicated and not fully understood. Epidemiological studies show that the risk of thrombo-embolic disease is less with lower oestrogen doses. The effect of COC on congenital deficiency of protein C needs further study
2. *Thrombotic and cardiovascular risks*
   (i) Venous thrombosis risk increased 3–6 times. Related to oestrogen dose. Correlated to smoking. Disappears when COC stops
   (ii) Haemorrhagic stroke — 2 times risk. Related to smoking and hypertension
   (iii) Thrombolytic stroke — 5 times risk. Not effected by smoking and hypertension
   (iv) Myocardial infarction risk. Risk times 2. Related to age and smoking, but COC not necessarily contra-indicated in women from 35 to 45 years if they do not smoke

(v) Mesenteric vascular ischaemia. Rare. Most of the data on which these risks are based involve higher dose COC

Women undergoing major elective surgery should use another form of contraception for 6 weeks before and 4 weeks after it. It is also not advisable to take the pill if one or both legs are immobilised in plaster casts.

Hypertension develops in about 5% of women within five years of commencing the combined pill. These should be stopped if, having had a normal blood pressure beforehand, it rises to or above 160 mmHg systolic and/or 95 mmHg diastolic on repeated readings.

Older women, and those with a past history or family history of hypertension, are at greater risk. Obesity and previous hypertension in pregnancy are not associated risks. If the BP rises or stays high after delivery this is probably due to underlying chronic vascular disease or essential hypertension unmasked by pregnancy. Patients with a history of pre-eclampsia can be tried on COC, but BP must be watched closely in the first few months.

Varicose veins may become more pronounced. Minor degrees of varicosities are not a contra-indication to oral contraceptives but severe degrees are.

3. *Hepatic effects*. There is a slightly increased risk of developing the rare hepatocellular adenoma and even rarer adenocarcinoma of the liver after prolonged use of the combined pill.

   Jaundice may arise in women taking the pill if they have:
   (i) Had intrahepatic cholestasis during pregnancy
   (ii) A history of chronic idiopathic jaundice (e.g. Dubin–Johnson or Rotor syndrome)
   (iii) Abnormal liver function as a residue of viral hepatitis

   The combined pill may accelerate the presentation of pre-existing gall-bladder disease but, in the long term does not increase the number of cases
4. *Psychological effects*. Steroidal contraceptives may reduce libido in some women both as a direct effect and by causing coital difficulties due to impairment of lubrication. In others libido is increased because the risk of an unwanted pregnancy is removed.

   The combined pill may be associated with episodes of depression. This can be due to lack of vitamin B6 (pyridoxine) and may respond to its prescription.

   The premenstrual syndrome is alleviated by the pill in many women.
5. *Post-pill amenorrhoea* — see p. 174
6. *Tumorogenic effects*. The suggestion of an increased risk of breast cancer among women taking the combined pill is

controversial. The balance of evidence suggests that the use of COC by mature women does not increase the risk, but there is serious doubt about its use for more than four years at a young age in relation to breast cancer developing before 36 years. If such a risk exists it can be minimised by using the lowest effective doses of oestrogen and progestogen.

Cervical intraepithelial neoplasia may be indirectly associated in that it is related to sexual activity which may be facilitated by oral contraception. There may be some direct effect of COC on carcinoma of the cervix, but this has to be set against the strongly protective effect against carcinoma of endometrium and ovary (see Benefits).

7. *Chronic inflammatory bowel disease*. The risk of Crohn's disease may be doubled in COC takers. The effect on ulcerative colitis is less clear.

In summary, the risk/benefit balance must be weighed for each woman taking into account the prevailing risks in each particular population. For instance, the balance will be much altered where the risks of pregnancy and childbirth are high and/or the cardiovascular risk is low.

Drug interactions

1. *Enzyme-inducing drugs* may reduce the effect of oestrogens and progestogens. They include most anti-convulsants (not sodium valproate), rifampicin, griseofulvin, phenylbutazone, spironolactone and some tranquillizers.
2. *Interference with gut flora* and the enterohepatic circulation of ethinyloestradiol can be caused by broad spectrum antibiotics (also by a vegetarian diet). Progestogens are not effected in this way.
   Large doses of VitC, and co-trimoxazole can raise oestrogen levels.

Conversely, the pill interferes with the action of warfarin and tricyclic drugs. The former is of no practical importance because if anticoagulants are necessary, the pill is contra-indicated.

Contra-indications to combined oral contraceptives

1. Absolute
   - (i) Previous arterial or venous thrombosis and especially if associated with coagulation tendency
   - (ii) Severe heart disease or pulmonary hypertension
   - (iii) Blood dyscrasias
   - (iv) In the presence of a malignant neoplasm, particularly carcinoma of the breast
   - (v) Chronic liver disease and following acute disease until liver function tests have been normal for three months
   - (vi) Liver adenoma

(vii) Severe hypertension
(viii) History of serious condition affected by sex steroids, e.g. pemphigoid gestations
(ix) Pregnancy
(x) Undiagnosed abnormal genital tract bleeding

2. Relative
(i) Oligo-amenorrhoea — investigate first and can then be prescribed
(ii) Women over 35 years of age who smoke
(iii) Latent or established diabetes
(iv) Cholelithiasis but can be used after cholecystecomy
(v) Renal disease
(vi) Obesity, if associated with other risk factors
(vii) Migraine — this becomes absolute if focal, or ergotamine is required for treatment
(viii) Sickle-cell disease: injectable progestogen better. Sickle-cell trait not a contra-indication
(x) Crohn's disease

3. Situations in which current use must be reviewed
(i) In face of elective surgery or immobilisation in a plaster cast
(ii) When the patient complains of cramps, pain or oedema of the legs
(iii) Sudden migraine attacks or unusual headaches
(iv) Severe chest pain
(v) Visual disturbance
(vi) Transient weakness of the limbs
(vii) If clinical or chemical evidence of diabetes develops
(viii) Viral hepatitis
(ix) Hypertension develops
(x) Depression develops
(xi) During antibiotic therapy } additional precautions must
(xii) Gastrointestinal upset } be taken

INTRA-UTERINE DEVICES

The ideal intrauterine device (IUD) should fulfil three criteria:
1. It must be effective
2. It must be easy to fit with minimal discomfort
3. It should remain in the uterine cavity until the woman wishes it removed

All devices presently available in the UK have copper wire round the stem (and transverse arms)

Timing of insertion

The best time is towards the end of menstruation but fitting can take place at any point in the cycle. After pregnancy the optimum time is 6 weeks after delivery. An IUD can be fitted at the time of suction termination of pregnancy but the optimum time is 1 to 2 weeks later because the risk of perforation is less.

Insertion of an IUD within 5 days of unprotected intercourse will act as a post-coital contraceptive.

Mode of action

The main effect is likely to depend on interference with events surrounding implantation and changes in utero-tubal environment may affect viability of ovum and sperm. The failure rate is between two and four pregnancies per 100 w.y. but with the newest devices carrying up to 380 mm^2 of copper this may be reduced to under 1 per 100 w.y.

Possible complications and side-effects of IUDs

1. Vaginal bleeding — a small amount of bleeding always follows insertion but spotting may occur for a few weeks.

   The first few menses will be heavier than previously and may remain so. None of a variety of remedies is entirely satisfactory for any length of time.

   A complaint of excessive menstrual loss is the commonest reason for changing to another form of contraception
2. Pain — some low abdominal pain or backache may follow insertion. Rarely it is severe and the patient may faint due to 'cervical shock'. Atropine 0.6 mg can be given i.v. if severe bradycardia occurs. The device may need to be removed.

   Dysmenorrhoea can be increased particularly if the woman is nulliparous
3. Vaginal discharge — may be temporary or persist. It arises from the endometrium as it reacts to the presence of a foreign body but symptomatic discharges must be investigated
4. Expulsion is most likely during the first month. About 50% of all expulsion take place within three months of insertion; after the first year very few are expelled. Among the associated factors are:
   (i) Young women of low parity
   (ii) Use of an inappropriate size or type of IUD
   (iii) The skill and experience of the person fitting the device
5. Lost threads. This may be due to:
   (i) Unrecognised expulsion
   (ii) Perforation of the uterus (see below)
   (iii) A normally sited device with the threads above the external os

   The woman may or may not be pregnant in each of the above circumstances.

   The site of the IUD can be checked by ultrasound. If the device is still *in utero* the threads may be retrieved using a MI-Mark Helix or a 3 to 4 mm Karman suction cannula.

Removal can be facilitated by the dilating effect on the cervix of ethinyloestradiol 50 μg b.d. for 5 days in mid-cycle. Embedded devices can be dissected out using a hysteroscope.

6. Perforation of the uterus occurs in about 1 in 1000 insertions. Most devices can be removed from the peritoneal cavity by laparoscopy or laparotomy through a small incision. Copper-bearing devices tend to form omental masses and adhesions, and should be removed promptly.
7. Infection is the most serious cause of morbidity associated with the use of an IUD. The major risk factor is the number of sexual partners of the woman and her partner. Monogamous women using a copper device have no increased risk. Age and gravidity are not risk factors other than in relation to the number of sexual partners.

   The infecting organisms can be aerobic or anaerobic, and the possible involvement of *Chlamydia* must be remembered (see p. 211). If infection is suspected, take appropriate swabs and consider antibiotic therapy. The IUD may need to be removed (if so send for bacteriological culture). Infections with *Actinomyces israeli* are a rare complication
8. Pregnancy complications. If the woman becomes pregnant with an IUD in place the risk of spontaneous abortion is higher than average, particularly if the device is left *in situ*. The device should therefore be removed if the threads are accessible.

   A major associated complication is second-trimester septic abortion (p. 15). Ectopic pregnancy is not prevented, but a direct cause and effect relationship between it and IUD use is difficult to demonstrate. Intrauterine candidal infection resulting in fetal death can rarely occur

Contra-indications to the use of an IUD

1. *Absolute*
   (i) Pregnancy
   (ii) Recent septic abortion
   (iii) Active pelvic inflammatory disease
   (iv) Congenital uterine anomaly
   (v) Abnormal uterine bleeding (investigate and correct)
   (vi) Carcinoma of cervix or endometrium
   (vii) Copper allergy or Wilson's disease
2. *Relative*
   (i) Multiple sexual partners
   (ii) Past history of STD
   (iii) Previous ectopic pregnancy
   (iv) Nulliparity
   (v) Menorrhagia
   (vi) Risk from bacteraemia, e.g. valvular heart disease, renal dialysis or transplant or immunosuppressive drugs

BARRIER CONTRACEPTION

Barrier contraceptives prevent live sperm from entering the cervical canal either by mechanical occlusion (caps and condoms) or by killing sperm (spermicides). Condoms are the most popular.

Caps include vaginal diaphragms, cervical caps, vault caps and vimules (see Suggested further reading).

The most commonly used is the diaphragm. It must be used in conjunction with spermicides, and it must be fitted before intercourse and removed 6 hours afterwards.

The use-effectiveness of these methods varies widely depending on the motivation of the couple, but the theoretical effectiveness of caps and condoms is high, with pregnancy rates as low as 2 per 100 woman-years.

Among recently married, similarly motivated couples 5% of condom-users and 4% of pill-users become pregnant during the first year of use.

Barrier methods have assumed great importance in the battle against the spread of HIV infection (see p. 101). They should therefore be discussed with ALL couples seeking contraceptive advice, even if they are using another method in addition.

SAFE-PERIOD METHODS

Among the methods used to detect the fertile and infertile phases in the cycle are:

1. Rhythm method
   The lengths of the previous 12 cycles are recorded and the time during which intercourse is to be avoided is between 18 and 11 days before the next period is due to begin. This method is not applicable if the cycle is very irregular, or after recent pregnancy, and may be affected by illness or emotional upset
2. Cyclical temperature changes
   These can be used in two main ways:
   (i) The couple abstain from sexual intercourse until 3 days after the temperature has risen
   (ii) Intercourse can take place in the early follicular phase and time of abstinence is determined by use of the calender and timing of the temperature rise.
3. Cervical mucus
   Cervical mucus becomes profuse and watery with a good spinnbarkeit at ovulation. Women can be taught to recognise these changes.

The popular 'sympto-thermal' method uses a combination of 2 and 3.

These methods are effective when used consistently by

highly-motivated couples, but even then it is reported that accidental pregnancy may occur in up to 14% of women using the sympto-thermal method for 2 years.

COITUS INTERRUPTUS

Male withdrawal is the oldest and most widely used method of contraception. It is simple, moderately effective and without serious side-effects (excluding pregnancy).

MALE AND FEMALE STERILISATION

Sterilisation in either partner is increasingly popular for birth control. The peak age in women is between 30 and 34 years. The popularity of this irreversible approach is due to the limitations of other, reversible, methods.

In counselling couples requesting sterilisation the following general points must be borne in mind:

1. The operation (either male or female) must be deemed to be irreversible
2. Alternative methods must have been considered fully
3. Sterilisation of either partner will not stabilise an insecure marriage
4. Agreement to sterilisation must *never* be a prior condition for agreement to undertake termination of pregnancy
5. Childbirth or abortion are stressful times and extra care must be taken to ensure that sterilisation at these times is appropriate
6. The small failure rate of all approaches must be explained
7. If postpartum sterilisation is being requested the couple must understand that the first year of life is the most dangerous for the infant and may therefore be advised to defer operation for some time, particularly if the child is sickly at birth
8. Written consent must be obtained from the person undergoing the operation and that of the other partner is advisable

Female sterilisation as a primary procedure

The current techniques in order of popularity are:

1. Laparoscopy — the Fallopian tubes are occluded by clips or bands or less commonly now bipolar diathermy. There is an associated mortality of about 8 per 100 000 laparoscopies
2. Mini-laparotomy — access to the tubes is by a proctoscope or similar instrument inserted through a small suprapubic incision
3. Laparotomy — the tubes should be divided and the ends separated

4. Posterior colpotomy — the tubes are approached through a small incision in the pouch of Douglas.

A comparison of male and female sterilisation

	Male	*Female*
Personnel required	1. Can be performed by one trained person 2. Training is relatively simple	1. Requires a team 2. A background of gynaecology or general surgery is necessary
Time and equipment	1. Quicker than for female 2. Local anaesthetic adequate 3. Very little equipment required	1. Longer than for male 2. More skilled and hazardous anaesthesia required 3. Equipment more sophisticated
Effect	Takes some time Re-canalisation more common	Immediate More difficult to reverse
Mortality	Nil when performed aseptically under local anaesthesia	About 8 per 100 000 operations
Short-term morbidity	Local infection and haematomas, epididymo-orchitis	Anaesthetic hazards, cardiac arrhythmias, infection, pain and haemorrhage
Longer-term morbidity	Auto-immune testicular damage suggested but not proven	Menorrhagia due to operation not proven

Additional points

1. If female sterilisation is to be by laparotomy, oral contraception should stop one month beforehand and adequate alternative contraception used
2. The failure rate of female sterilisation is between 0.2% and 1% depending on the type of operation and experience of the operator
3. Two sperm-free specimens should be obtained from a man who has undergone vasectomy before he can be deemed to be sterile. The first sperm-free specimen should be collected only after at least 12 postoperative ejaculations have taken place.

   If seminal examination is impossible due to lack of facilities or inability of the man to return for check-up provide him with 20 condoms to be used for every act of intercourse until they are used up

4. Reversibility. If the technique used for vasectomy is amenable to reversal, sperm will return to the ejaculate in about two-thirds of men, and about one-third of their partners will become pregnant.

Tubal re-anastomosis in women will restore fertility in between 50 and 70% of women, varying with the method of sterilisation and the experience of the operator. Ectopic pregnancy can be expected in about 8% of conceptions

CONTRACEPTIVE USAGE

It is estimated that, in 1983, about 75% of all women aged 18 to 44 used some form of contraception. The most popular methods were:

Oral contraception	28%
(50%of women aged 20 to 24)	
Sterilisation (male and female)	22%
Condom	13%
(40% of women aged 35 to 44)	

Of the 25% not using contraception about half were at risk of pregnancy and less than 10% of the total wished to become pregnant. No more recent national figures are available. A rise in condom use in response to HIV risk in to be expected.

SUGGESTED FURTHER READING

Filshie M, Guillebaud J 1989 Contraception: science and practice. Butterworth, London

Loudon N 1985 Handbook of family planning. Churchill Livingstone, Edinburgh

McEwan J 1985 Hormonal methods of contraception and their adverse effect. In: Studd J (ed) Progress in obstetrics and gynaecology. Churchill Livingstone, Edinburgh, Vol 5, p 259

Pelvic infections

PELVIC INFLAMMATORY DISEASE (PID)

Primary — an infection which ascends from the lower genital tract due to:

1. Sexually transmitted diseases (STDs) caused by organisms such as *N. gonorrhoeae*, *C. trachomatis*, *M. hominis* and *U. urealyticum*. PID is the most common serious complication of STDs, and these organisms cause more than 70% of all cases
2. Ascent of endogenous vaginal and perianal flora (usually anaerobic organisms)
3. Iatrogenic e.g. D & C., HSG, tubal insufflation, termination of pregnancy, insertion of an IUD. This comprises about 15% of all cases (0.5% post TOP)
4. After delivery or miscarriage

Secondary — an infection caused by:

1. Direct spread from near by pelvic organs (most often the appendix)

or

2. Associated with other diseases e.g. schistosomiasis or filariasis

This constitutes less than 1% of all cases.

Epidemiology

Pelvic inflammatory disease is rare in women who are not sexually active. The overall incidence is 10–13 per 1000 women of reproductive age, with a peak of 20 per 1000 in the 15–24 year age group.

Among the factors which have contributed to the increased incidence of PID are:

An increased world population
Populations have tended to become urbanised
Attitudes to sex have changed, and the age of commencing sexual activity has fallen
Travel has increased, and casual sexual encounters are much more common away from home

Bacteriology
There are many infective agents capable of causing PID. A gonococcal infection may pave the way for anaerobic organisms or may lead to tubal damage and increased susceptibility to subsequent infection by organisms of usually low pathogenicity. In recurrent PID the proportion of non-gonococcal cases increases by 50%, suggesting a decreased ability to combat subsequent infection.

The major organisms involved are:

1. *Neisseria gonorrhoeae* (see p. 253) — isolated from the cervices of between 10 and 70% of women with salpingitis. Gonococcal salpingitis tends to occur within the first half of the menstrual cycle.
   As many as 60% of women with gonorrhoea have no symptoms for months or even years.
   Up to 10% of men may be symptomless carriers.
   The organism is becoming increasingly resistant to penicillin.
   Diagnosis is by direct inoculation of cervical, urethral and rectal and throat swabs onto Thayer–Martin plates
2. *Chlamydia trachomatis* causes more than half of all cases of PID in women under 25 years of age and is a potent cause of tubal occlusion because the damage done is out of proportion to its clinical severity. It is frequently associated with postpartum endometritis and is the recognised cause of the uncommon Fitz-Hugh–Curtis syndrome of perihepatitis.
   This organism also causes non-specific urethritis and lymphogranuloma venereum
3. Anaerobic organisms most frequently gain access from the lower genital tract in women whose uterus and tubes have already been affected by sexually transmitted organisms. The anaerobes most commonly involved are *Bacteroides* spp (especially *B. fragilis*) *Peptococcus* and *Peptostreptococcus*. They occur regularly in the cervical flora of healthy women so they are of doubtful significance if found in cervical swab cultures. If swabs are to be taken it is probably best done at laparoscopy (see below)
4. *Mycoplasma hominis* and *Ureaplasma urealyticum* may be responsible for 10 to 15% of cases in women under the age of 25 years. *M. hominis* tends to cause parametritis rather than salpingitis. Posterior fornix swabs will show if these organisms are at least present in the lower genital tract; otherwise direct swabbing of the tubes at laparoscopy is necessary
5. Other organisms which have been implicated include coliforms, *H. influenzae* and streptococci (Groups B and D) but they are usually secondary to a primary gonococcal infection. It has also been suggested that viruses such as

herpes simplex may play a role but there is no direct evidence of this

Sequelae

1. *Chronic pelvic pain* — 20% of patients will suffer from this long-term problem and of these 60–70% will be infertile and/or have dyspareunia
2. *Heavy and irregular menses* due to chronic pelvic inflammation.
3. *Subfertility* results from 15 to 20% of cases
4. *Ectopic pregnancy*. PID increases the risk by seven-to ten-fold

Diagnosis

Clinical features of acute PID

The classical clinical features are:

1. Acute pelvic pain
2. Pyrexia 38–39°C
3. Tender adnexae (often with palpable unilateral or bilateral swellings)
4. Raised white cell count and ESR
5. There may be some menstrual irregularity

Diagnostic accuracy, if only the above criteria are relied on, may be as low as 35% and is certainly no better than 65%.

Among the conditions most frequently causing false-positive or false-negative errors in differential diagnosis are:

Acute appendicitis
Endometriosis
Ectopic pregnancy
Corpus luteum haemorrhage
Ovarian cysts
Inflammatory conditions of other organs

In addition, although the above clinical criteria are associated with patients with acute PID when looked at as a group, the fact that they can be present in up to 20% of women with no pelvic pathology means that they cannot be relied on as the sole means of diagnosis.

Laparoscopy is the most reliable method for diagnosis but it has its hazards. For positive diagnosis all of the following features must be present:

1. Erythema of Fallopian tubes
2. Oedema and swelling of tubes
3. Seropurulent exudate on the surface of the tube from the fimbriated end

The condition is *mild* if these criteria are present but the tubes are mobile and patent; *moderate* if the findings are more florid, the tubes are not mobile and their patency is uncertain; and *severe* if a tubo-ovarian mass or masses are present.

The inflammation is usually but not invariably bilateral.
Swabs can be taken for culture at laparoscopy from the Fallopian tubes or the pouch of Douglas.
Peritoneal fluid can also be cultured.

Treatment of acute PID

Antibiotic therapy

The rapidity with which antibiotics are prescribed depends on the clinical severity of the condition and initial choice is usually empirical. If specific organisms are cultured against which the prescribed antibiotic is not effective, or there is no improvement in the patient's signs and symptoms within 48 hours of commencing antibiotic therapy, the choice of drugs will need to be reviewed. The following are among the antibiotics most relevant to the treatment of acute PID bearing in mind the most likely infecting organisms:

1. *The penicillins.* The *ampicillins* (ampicillin, amoxycillin and talampicillin) are not particularly useful because they have no activity against beta-lactamase-producing *E. coli.* They are also ineffective against *Pseudomonas aeruginosa* and *Bacteroides fragilis.*

   The combination ot the beta-lactamase inhibitor, clavulanic acid and amoxycillin can overcome this problem.

   Mezlocillin and *azlocillin* are parenteral preparations related to ampicillin. They have a broad spectrum of activity including *Klebsiella, Proteus* spp, *B. fragilis, Strep. faecalis* and *P. aeruginosa.* They are also highly active against gonococci and act synergistically with aminoglycosides against certain Gram-negative bacilli. Their use is best reserved for severe infections, but they are not stable to beta-lactamases.

   Mecillinam and its oral analogue, *pivmecillinam,* are most active against Gram-negative organisms. They act synergistically with ampicillin and some cephalosporins. They too are hydrolysed by beta-lactamase-producing organisms
2. *Cephalosporins.* Most of the new generation of cephalosporins and cephalexin are active against coliforms, *Klebsiella* and *Proteus mirabilis,* gonococci, among other organisms. They are not effective against *P. aeruginosa.* Cefuroxime is stable to the action of many beta-lactamases, and is highly active against *N. gonorrhoeae* and *H. influenzae.* It must be given parenterally.

   Cefoxitin is also stable to beta-negative-lactamases and is highly effective against Gram-negative organisms (except for *P. aeruginosa*) and most strains of *B. fragilis.* It too can be given by injection

3. *Tetracyclines* remain the treatment of choice for chlamydial and mycoplasma infections. Their use is contra-indicated in pregnant women and growing children
4. *Erythromycin* has a similar antibacterial spectrum to penicillin and is, therefore, useful in penicillin-allergic patients. It is active against many penicillin-resistant staphylococci, gut anaerobes, chlamydia and mycoplasmas
5. *Aminoglycosides*. Gentamicin is still a useful parenteral antibiotic because of its action against most Gram-negative bacteria. It is inactive against anaerobes.

   The newer drugs outlined above are tending to displace gentamicin from its previous pre-eminence in severe infections
6. *Metronidazole* is invaluable in the treatment of infections due to *Bacteroides* spp, *Clostridium*, and many anaerobic streptococci. It is well absorbed after oral or rectal administration and should form at least part of the treatment in most cases.

   From the above resumé it should be possible to develop a rational policy for the use of antibiotics in PID as long as the drugs are used in therapeutic doses for an adequate length of time.

Surgery

The main role of surgery in the management of acute PID is after rupture of a tubo-ovarian abscess and to drain a pyosalpinx. Adnexal masses over 8 cm in diameter and bilateral tubo-ovarian abscesses tend not to respond to antibiotic therapy.

Chronic pelvic inflammatory disease

Pathology

1. Peritubal adhesions — the more vascular they are the more virulent have the infections been
2. Tubal occlusion and distortion. If both the distal and proximal ends of the tubes are blocked a pyosalpinx forms. As the infection subsides this becomes a hydrosalpinx. In the most severe forms it is typically retort-shaped
3. The ovary is often surrounded by dense adhesions and its substance may be destroyed to a greater or lesser extent depending on the severity of the infection

Clinical features

The patient classically complains of:

1. Heavy and irregular menses
2. Dysmenorrhoea
3. Dyspareunia

4. Chronic pelvic pain
5. Infertility

There may also be chronic vaginal discharge.

The uterus is tender and often fixed in retroversion. It may be displaced to one side by a pelvic mass. The adnexae are tender and may feel thickened.

Differential diagnosis
The condition which most closely mimics chronic PID is endometriosis.

Management
The feature which marks out this condition more than any other is its chronicity. It may be temporarily abated by conservative measures such as courses of antibiotics and short-wave diathermy to the pelvis but it is not cured by any of them.

Ultimately the drastic remedy of pelvic clearance may be the only one which will afford the unfortunate woman relief.

The results from surgery to increase fertility in the face of chronic PID are generally disappointing (see p. 196)

SUGGESTED FURTHER READING

Tindall V R 1990 Jeffcoate's principles of gynaecology. 5th edn. Butterworth, London

The management of pain

Definition
Pain is an unpleasant sensation arising from stimulation of specific nerve endings, transmitted through more or less specific central nervous pathways to higher centres in the brain mainly located in areas which subserve emotion.

Pain, emotion and personality are therefore inextricably linked.

PELVIC PAIN

Pelvic and lower abdominal pain are common complaints in gynaecology clinics. Our ability to help patients with chronic pelvic pain is poor once major organic causes have been excluded. This is as much a commentary on the doctor as the patient.

Aetiology
The following is a guide to some causes of acute and chronic pelvic pain.

	Acute pain	*Chronic pain*
Physiological	Ovulation pain	Mild dysmenorrhoea
Congenital	(Meckel's diverticulum)	Haematocolpos
Traumatic	Coitus injury to genital tract	As for dyspareunia Postsurgery adhesions
Infective		
Gynaecological	Vaginitis Acute pelvic inflammatory disease	Chronic pelvic inflammatory disease Pyosalpinges
Non-gynaecological	Urinary tract infection Appendicitis	Diverticulitis Irritable bowel syndrome

	Acute pain	Chronic pain
Neoplastic	Accident to ovarian cyst Degeneration of a fibroid	
Hormonal		Endometriosis
Mechanical	Hernia (inguinal or femoral). Bowel obstruction Prolapsed intervertebral disc	Utero-vaginal prolapse Orthopaedic conditions
Vascular		Pelvic congestion possibly due to dilated pelvic veins
Metabolic	Ureteric calculus	Rare conditions such as porphyria
Pregnancy-associated	Ectopic pregnancy Inevitable abortion Labour Red degeneration of a fibroid	Tension on adhesions (?)

Psychological
Among the factors which effect the perception of pain are the following:

1. *Sociocultural factors*
   Age (perception increased in very young and elderly)
   Race
   Education (understanding reduces perception)
   IQ
   Family and neighbourhood experiences
2. *Psychological factors*
   Previous experience
   Anxiety increases perception
   Excitement or aggression decreases perception
   Explanation decreases perception
   The provision of pain relief
3. *Psychosocial factors*
   Sexual problems
   Marital dysharmony
   Problems with children (particularly infants and teenagers)
   Financial difficulties

Investigation

History

A full history is vital and must aim to define:

1. Site and radiation of pain
2. Duration and nature of onset
3. Character of the pain (sharp, dull, etc.)
4. Periodicity of the pain (constant, intermittent)
5. Intensity of the pain (e.g. effect on sleep, work, play)
6. Relationship to: menses, micturition, food, movement, coitus, defaecation, posture
7. What improves it and effect of any analgesics (to be specified)
8. Psychological status e.g. any family problems or sexual difficulties

Examination

1. General appearance (tense, anxious?)
2. General and pelvic examination — *Note*: the bladder must be empty

Further investigation

Expensive and potentially hazardous investigations must not be ordered merely as a routine.
Among the investigations which may be helpful as indicated by the history and examination are:

1. Pelvic ultrasonography
2. Straight X-ray of abdomen
3. Excretion urography (IVP)
4. Barium meal with follow-through or enema (after IVP to avoid residual barium obscuring view)
5. EUA and laparoscopy
6. Sigmoidoscopy

Subsequent management

Any organic lesion can be treated appropriately. If no specific cause is immediately apparent obtain more information from the patient's general practitioner and herself (gently) about possible contributory psychosexual, emotional, financial or social problems.

It is very difficult to deal adequately with the woman complaining of chronic pain without obvious cause in the hospital setting. She must not be given the impression that the doctors feel she is imagining it. A psychosomatic pain is as real as any other.

Some patients use the subjective nature of pain for their own ends because they know that no one can say categorically that they are not suffering.

Principles of management

1. Treat underlying physical causes
2. Attempt to provide the patient with insight into the impact her emotions have on perception of pain
3. Aim to make the pain tolerable in the first instance by simple measures such as sympathy, promoting positive aspects of the patient's personality or antidepressant drugs (if the woman is depressed)
4. Analgesics. Aspirin and paracetamol are still the basis of any treatment regimen. The drug should be taken in anticipation of the pain rather than when it has built up. A fortified aspirin or paracetamol compound should be tried next if the above are not adequate, e.g. propoxyphene with paracetamol; codeine or dihydrocodeine. Laxatives will usually be necessary also because of the constipative effects of codeine and its derivatives. Non-steroidal anti-inflammatory agents are sometimes useful particularly for dysmenorrhoea
5. Psychiatric help may be valuable in some cases

PAIN RELIEF IN ADVANCED MALIGNANT DISEASE

Principles

Aim to keep the patient both free of pain and fully alert.

Assessment

1. Treatment varies according to the cause of the pain; use body chart to record sites of pain and their probable mechanism
2. Because a person has cancer, it does not mean that the malignant process is necessarily the cause of the pain
3. Many patients require a combination of drug and non-drug measures, e.g. radiation for bone pain, nerve blocks for nerve compression pain

Choice of analgesics

1. Establish a simple, practical analgesic 'league table':
   Non-narcotic — aspirin (alt. paracetamol)
   Weak narcotic — codeine (alt. DHC. d-propoxyphene)
   Strong narcotic — morphine (alt. papaveretum, diamorphine)
2. Avoid pentazocine, pethidine and dextromoromide (Palfium)
3. Methadone should be used with caution, particularly in the elderly and debilitated
4. The use of a narcotic analgesic is dictated by intensity of pain and not by brevity of prognosis. 'Morphine exists to be given, not merely to be withheld'

Use of analgesics
Oral medication is normally possible. When injections are necessary, use freeze-dried ampoules of diamorphine.
Persistent pain requires preventive therapy. This means that analgesics should be given regularly and prophylactically: 'as required' medication is both irrational and inhumane.
Doses should be determined on an individual basis; the right dose is that which gives relief for at least three, preferably 4 or more hours.
Adjuvant medication is the rule rather than the exception.
Laxatives are almost always necessary, an anti-emetic commonly so.
Patients with metastatic bone pain often benefit by concurrent use of an aspirin-like drug: those with nerve compression pain may be helped by *prednisolone.*
If very anxious, an anxiolytic such as diazepam should be tried; if depressed, an antidepressive.
The perception of pain requires both attention and consciousness. Diversional therapy — people to talk to, activities to attend, etc. — is of great value.
Tolerance is not usually a practical problem.
Rightly used, psychological dependence (addiction) does not occur.
Physical dependence does not prevent the downward adjustment of the dose of a narcotic analgesic should the pain ameliorate.
Neither diamorphine nor morphine is the panacea for terminal pain. Their use does not guarantee automatic success, particularly if the psychological component of pain is ignored.

Re-assessment
Relief of pain should be assessed in relation to comfort achieved:
1. During the night
2. In the daytime at rest
3. On movement

Re-assessment remains a continuing necessity. Old pains may get worse and new ones may develop.

SUGGESTED FURTHER READING

Hobbs J T 1990 The pelvic congestion syndrome. British Journal of Hospital Medicine 43: 200–206

Disorders of micturition

URINARY INCONTINENCE

20 to 30% of women over the age of 65 years are said to suffer from a significant degree of urinary incontinence.

Definitions

1. *Stress incontinence*
   (i) Symptom: the involuntary loss of a small amount of urine during exercise, coughing, sneezing, etc.
   (ii) Sign: involuntary urine loss is observed when abdominal pressure is increased
   (iii) Condition: the involuntary loss of urine when the intravesical pressure exceeds the maximum urethral pressure in the absence of detrusor activity
2. *Urge incontinence* is the involuntary loss of urine associated with a strong desire to micturate.
   (i) Motor urgency associated with uninhibited detrusor contractions
   (ii) Sensory urgency due to irritative lesions (e.g. cystitis, calculus, tumour) in which the detrusor is stable
3. *Reflex incontinence* is the involuntary loss of urine due to abnormal spinal reflex activity in the absence of the sensation to micturate
4. *Overflow incontinence* is the involuntary loss of urine when the intravesical pressure exceeds maximum urethral pressure due to bladder distension and in the absence of detrusor activity
5. *True incontinence* is the involuntary loss of urine due to a defect in the anatomical integrity of the urinary tract

Investigation

Past history

(i) Past medical and surgical history e.g. STD; polio; surgery to spine or genito-urinary tract; cerebral, spinal or pelvic trauma
(ii) Gynaecological and obstetric history (particularly of rapid or slow labours, large infants)

(iii) Previous urological complaints (e.g. enuresis, urinary infections, haematuria)
(iv) Family history (e.g. enuresis, diabetes)
(v) Social history (e.g. drug abuse, excessive alcohol ingestion or cigarette smoking)

Present complaint
(i) Duration and whether continuous or intermittent
(ii) If incontinent type, amount of loss, degree of social inconvenience
(iii) Urgency of micturition?
(iv) Voiding difficulties? — initiation; stream; termination
(v) Frequency of micturition — diurnal and nocturnal
(vi) Incidence of urinary infections

Symptomatic guide to detrusor activity
The following symptoms suggest that the detrusor is stable or unstable.

Stable	*Unstable*
Only symptom is stress incontinence	Urgency and urge incontinence
Micturition normal	Frequency and nocturia
Urine loss small	Urine loss great
Able to interrupt flow*	Unable to interrupt flow*

* Many women do not know whether they can or cannot interrupt flow.

Pelvic examination to demonstrate incontinence, utero-vaginal prolapse and detect any other pelvic pathology. Note oestrogenisation of the vaginal wall, the ability to contract the pelvic floor and scarring from any previous surgery.

Note. Prolapse and incontinence are not directly related: there is a higher incidence of detrusor instability in patients with incontinence and prolapse than in those without prolapse.

Urine microscopy and culture are compulsory.

Urodynamic tests
1. Tests of urine flow will differentiate abnormal from normal voiding and can evaluate the results of surgical treatment of the bladder neck
2. Cystometry primarily tests the reservoir function of the bladder. Intravesical and abdominal (*rectal*) pressures should be measured simultaneously. By subtractiing the latter from the former intrinsic (detrusor) bladder pressure can be determined. Cystometry should be performed with the patient supine then erect because detrusor instability may not be detected in the supine position. A urethral pressure profile can also be performed at this time

3. Micturition cystourethrography is helpful in assessing the anatomical relationship of the urethra, urethro-vesical junction and bladder base, and in noting the sign of stress incontinence.
   X-ray pictures are taken at rest, during coughing or bearing down, and at the beginning, middle and end of micturition
4. Video-cystourethrography combines measurement of bladder pressure, urine flow and volume with (3) above. It is especially suitable for the assessment of detrusor instability and neurological disturbances.
5. Transvaginal endosonography can elucidate the anatomy of the bladder neck

Among the indications for urodynamic investigations are:
The combined symptoms of stress and urge incontinence
Stress incontinence with frequency and nocturia
A complaint of perpetual wetness
Failed surgery for similar complaint
Adult enuresis
Abnormal neurological signs
An intravenous urogram will help to exclude congenital anomalies, calculi or ureteric fistulae. Cystoscopy is not routinely carried out but useful information can be gained from it, and it is compulsory if the patient has had haematuria or there is suspicion of a pelvic mass.

For other investigations see Suggested further reading.

STRESS INCONTINENCE

Aetiology

The traditional teaching has been that loss of the posterior urethro-vesical angle is the main factor allowing stress incontinence to occur. However, urodynamic investigations have made it clear that, although loss of the posterior angle can be due to an intrinsic weakness of the bladder neck it may also arise because of contraction of an unstable detrusor.

Continence in the female is achieved because the urethro-vesical junction and proximal urethra are above the pelvic floor muscles and therefore intra-abdominal structures. Any rise in intra-abdominal pressure is transmitted equally to the bladder and proximal urethra which preserves the pressure gradient and maintains the positive urethral closure pressure (see section (a) in the Figure).

Genuine stress incontinence will tend to occur when an alteration in position of the bladder neck in relation to the pelvic flow (section (b) in the Figure) means that most of the urethra is below it.

Any increase in intra-abdominal pressure will increase intravesical but not urethral pressure. The former will exceed the

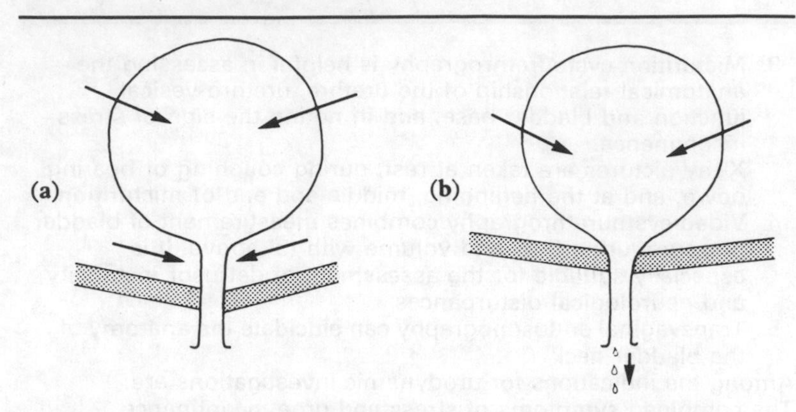

latter (i.e. there is a negative urethral closure pressure) and a small amount of urine will be lost.

These changes may or may not be accompanied by a cystocele.

Other features found in association with stress incontinence are funnelling of the bladder neck on exertion or straining (without detrusor activity) and a short functional length of the urethra.

The position of the bladder neck and efficiency of the distal voluntary sphincter mechanism may be affected adversely by childbirth, pelvic surgery, and postmenopausal hormonal changes. The defect may however be congenital such as a very short urethra, the 'relaxed bladder neck' syndrome and female epispadias when the bladder neck is deficient.

Treatment of stress incontinence

1. *Physiotherapy*. Pelvic floor exercises are useful prophylaxis after childbirth, but only partial success can be expected with established stress incontinence
2. *Drug therapy*. Genuine stress incontinence is not amenable to treatment with anticholinergic drugs but correction of oestrogen deficiency in postmenopausal women may be beneficial
3. *Surgery* aims to achieve some or all of the following effects.
   (i) Restoration of the position of the proximal urethra as an intra-abdominal structure
   (ii) Increase in the urethral closure pressure
   (iii) Increase in functional urethral length
   (iv) Increase in support to bladder neck and therefore its competence

Anterior colporrhaphy is the traditional gynaecological remedy but, although it is appropriate for the management of anterior vaginal wall prolapse, its role in curing stress incontinence is being questioned. Cure rates of 50 to 60% have been reported, but this is less than for other procedures in similarly experienced hands.

Primary suprapubic procedures are reported to have success rates of 80 to 90%. Among them are:

(i) Urethropexy by the Marshall–Marchetti and Krantz technique. Elevation of the bladder neck is achieved by suturing the para-urethral and para-vesical tissues to cartilage of the symphysis pubis or periosteum of the pubic ramus
(ii) Colposuspension by the Burch technique in which the bladder neck and anterior vaginal wall are elevated by suturing the para-vaginal fascia to the ipsilateral ileo-pectineal ligament
(iii) Endoscopic bladder neck suspension (Stamey procedure) — not best suited to elderly women
(iv) Urethro-vesical slings using either muscular or fascial strips or Mersilene gauze. These procedures are complicated to perform and require a combined vaginal and abdominal approach

Full details of these procedures can be found under Suggested further reading

4. *Mechanical devices.* If uterovaginal prolapse is a significant accompaniment of the stress incontinence and if the woman is not fit or refuses surgery a vaginal ring pessary may be of some benefit (see p. 236).

   Electrical stimulation may improve stress incontinence but electrical devices have only a relatively small role in the treatment of this condition usually in those awaiting or unfit for surgery.

   Inflatable devices have been developed which exert pressure within the vagina to elevate the bladder neck and they are preferable to electrical devices and are indicated in similar circumstances.

   An implantable artificial sphincter can be inserted, an inflatable cuff being used to occlude the bladder neck
5. *Urinary diversion procedures* may ultimately be necessary in a few patients in whom all other methods have failed. The construction of an ileal conduit is the usual method

DETRUSOR INSTABILITY

Aetiology

The cause of primary instability of the detrusor remains unknown. Some few cases are secondary to or associated with:

1. An upper motor neurone lesion e.g. multiple sclerosis
2. Inflammation — this tends to produce exacerbation of an existing instability rather than produce the condition itself
3. Lack of oestrogen in menopausal women
4. Bladder outflow obstruction. This is rare in women

Primary detrusor instability may be a variant of normal bladder function because it is the natural state in all infants and about 10% of the population never develop stable bladder function.

It is perhaps not surprising therefore that treatment of primary detrusor instability is so unsatisfactory. Among the suggested modes of treatment are:

1. *Bladder training* is a simple approach with as good or better results than any other remedy. The patient is admitted to hospital to assess the extent of her problem. She is then instructed to pass urine by the clock during the day. The interval starts at, minimally, 20 minutes and gradually increases. When good progress is being made she can return home to continue the bladder drill at home.
   It can be used in conjunction with drug therapy
2. *Drug therapy*. Drugs with anticholinergic activity may be beneficial usually only for as long as they are taken. Hormone replacement therapy (see p. 286) may be needed in some women
3. *Surgery* is not indicated

GENITOURINARY FISTULAE

1. Uretero-vaginal fistulae usually follow hysterectomy (particularly radical surgery)
2. High vesico-vaginal fistulae can follow lower segment Caesarean section, uterine rupture, hysterectomy or radiotherapy for cervical carcinoma. The ureteric orifices may be near the edge.
3. Mid-vaginal vesico-vaginal fistulae may be caused by pressure necrosis after prolonged obstructed labour or colporrhaphy fistulae. These are the commonest and are mostly due either to pressure necrosis or trauma by rotational forceps
4. Peri-urethral
5. Urethral fistulae. These may occasionally be so large as to virtually destroy the whole urethra and the bladder neck

Some defects will close spontaneously and all will heal to some extent if given enough time. Even if spontaneous closure does not occur surgery should be deferred to allow maximum tissue healing. The approximate intervals will depend on the cause, for example:

Surgical trauma;	about 10 weeks
Obstructed labour;	about 3 to 6 months
Radiation;	may be up to a year or more

Pre-operative management

In addition to attending to the patient's general health among the pre-operative investigations which should be carried out are urine culture and sensitivity, intravenous urography, cystoscopy and assessment under anaesthesia. If the fistula is associated with radiotherapy for neoplasm a biopsy of the edge should be taken to exclude residual tumour activity.

Operative closure
Technical details of closure are found in Suggested further reading, but among the important points are:

1. All but the simplest cases should be referred to centres or surgeons with special expertise
2. Most urethro-vaginal and vesico-vaginal fistulae can be repaired vaginally by dissection and repair in layers
3. The bladder wall closure must be watertight
4. The first attempt at repair has the best chance of success. Over 70% of fistulae can be closed at the first attempt, falling to about 30% if three or more repairs have previously been attempted.
5. Continuous catheter drainage is necessary for a minimum of 10 days (up to 3 weeks for radiation fistulae). The drainage system should be closed.

In any subsequent pregnancy all deliveries should be by elective Caesarean section.

VOIDING DIFFICULTIES

The urethral syndrome

Definition
Recurrent attacks of frequent and painful micturition not associated with any significant abnormality in the urinary tract and irrespective of the presence or absence of bacteriuria.

It is used synonymously with 'recurrent cystitis'.

Aetiology
Significant bacteriuria (>10^6 organisms/ml) is present in only about half of the cases.

1. *Infective causes.* It is frequently associated with lack of personal hygiene. There may be accompanying vulvo-vaginitis. The commonest infective agents are normal bowel flora. Among the others are *T. vaginalis, N. gonorrhoeae* and *C. trachomatis.*

   Tuberculosis of the bladder is a rare cause.
2. *Gynaecological causes.* Associated gynaecological symptoms and signs are common but their relevance in this condition is often assumed rather than proven e.g. cervical ectropion. The method of contraception may be important. Postmenopausal oestrogen deficiency is a definite cause.
3. *Chemical or allergic reactions.* This may be due to soaps,

douches, deodorants, contraceptive foam or anti-oxidants in condoms. It can also arise by wearing nylon underwear or tights.
4. *Sexual causes.* It can be due to too frequent or clumsy intercourse or masturbation with a foreign body. Its occasional association with first intercourse has caused the term 'honeymoon cystitis' to arise.
5. *Psychological causes.* Anxiety and neuroticism are not infrequent associations. Which is cause and which effect is not always entirely clear.
6. *Bladder problems.* Bladder outlet obstruction is much rarer in women than it is in men. It occurs in under 8% of women with the urethral syndrome.
   Detrusor instability is present in over 25% of cases. A bladder tumour is a rare cause but it must be suspected if there is haematuria
7. *Other causes.* Multiple sclerosis may rarely present in this fashion.

Clinical assessment
A full history is vital. Haematuria requires full investigation. Women with continuous and persistent frequency and dysuria are more likely to have a bladder lesion. A full gynaecological assessment is vital.

Investigation
1. Routine urine testing for protein, glucose and blood
2. Urine microscopy and culture
3. Cystoscopy contributes little if carried out routinely but is necessary in the presence of haematuria
4. Excretion urography (IVP) is indicated when urinary symptoms involve more than the lower urinary tract, haematuria is present, or recurrent urinary infections are occurring
5. Urodynamic testing is not recommended routinely

Treatment
1. Encourage simple perineal and introital hygiene but not antiseptic douching or bathing
2. A high fluid intake often helps — i.e. at least 5 litres for 24 to 48 hours. Potassium citrate and sodium bicarbonate may help also
3. Advise the use of cotton rather than nylon clothing
4. Treat any associated vulvo-vaginitis or vaginal discharge
5. Commence antibiotic therapy if symptoms do not subside within 48 hours of commencing a high fluid intake. The length of therapy depends on the patient's past history

6. Use hormone replacement therapy (in 3-month courses) in menopausal women
7. Consider urethral dilatation if symptoms persist or recur at frequent intervals. It is carried out under general anaesthetic and only the distal part of the urethra needs to be dilated (up to 35 Charrière gauge)
8. If a bladder neck obstruction can be demonstrated unequivocally endoscopic incision of the bladder neck can be carried out

An optimistic attitude and positive approach to treatment is important because there is often an understandably large functional overlay in these patients.

SUGGESTED FURTHER READING

Kelly J 1983 Vesico-vaginal fistulae. In: Studd J (ed) Progress in obstetrics and gynaecology. Churchill Livingstone, Edinburgh, Vol 3, p 324

Malvern J 1984 Incontinence of urine in women. In: Chamberlain G (ed) Contemporary gynaecology. Butterworths, London, p 200

Raz S 1985 Gynaecological urology. Clinics in obstetrics and gynaecology. Saunders, London, Vol 12, No. 2

Tindall V R 1990 Jeffcoate's principles of gynaecology. 5th edn. Butterworths, London

Uterine displacement and utero-vaginal prolapse

RETROVERSION

Mobile retroversion of the uterus is a variant of normal occurring in over 25% of women. It is usually asymptomatic and too many gynaecological symptoms have been attributed to it in the past. Backache is more frequently due to other conditions. An associated positioning of the ovaries in the pouch of Douglas may be a cause of dyspareunia.

Retroversion is not a cause of subfertility.

An acutely retroverted gravid uterus may become 'impacted' in the pelvis as the uterus enlarges. Acute retention of urine may result.

Mobile retroversion can be temporarily corrected by insertion of a Hodge pessary into the vagina.

Fixed retroversion is most frequently due to pelvic inflammatory disease (p. 219) or endometriosis (p. 183). The associated symptoms and signs and the management depend on the underlying disease.

Ventrosuspension by laparoscopy or laparotomy shortens the round ligaments by suturing them to the rectus sheath. It is seldom indicated.

UTERO-VAGINAL PROLAPSE

Definition

The downward displacement of the uterus and/or vagina towards or through the introitus. The bladder, urethra, rectum and bowel may be secondarily involved.

The uterus and vagina are mainly supported by the *levatores ani* muscles of the pelvic floor which form a downwards and forwards sloping gutter slung around the midline structures. The three components of the *levatores ani* are *ischio-coccygeus*, *ilio-coccygeus*, and *pubo-coccygeus*.

Prolapse has three degrees of severity:

First degree: descent of the cervix, to the introitus

Second degree: descent of the cervix, but not the whole uterus,

through the introitus
Third degree (procidentia): descent of the cervix and the whole uterus through the introitus.

Aetiology

Attenuation of the support mechanisms may occur as a result of:

1. *Childbirth* — prolapse is uncommon in nulliparous women. Prolonged labours with difficult vaginal deliveries may predispose to the development of prolapse subsequently. Precipitate labour may indicate some degree of deficiency of the pelvic floor which may later express itself as prolapse
2. *Postmenopausal atrophy*
3. *Chronic elevation of intra-abdominal pressure* due, for example, to obesity or a chronic cough

VAGINAL WALL PROLAPSE

A prolapse of the lowest third of the anterior vaginal wall involves the urethra and is therefore termed a *urethrocoele*.

In the upper two-thirds the bladder is involved and it is, therefore, a *cystocoele*.

A prolapse of the pouch of Douglas is an *enterocoele* because the hernial sac contains gut or omentum.

A prolapse of the posterior vaginal wall brings the rectum with it and is therefore a *rectocoele* which is not to be confused with prolapse of the rectal mucosa through the anus.

Symptoms

1. A feeling of 'something coming down'
2. Awareness of a lump protruding from the vulva
3. Discomfort and backache
4. Stress incontinence may occur because the urethra lies caudal to the pelvic floor (see p. 228) and not primarily because of loss of the posterior urethro-vesical angle
5. Urinary retention or difficulty with defaecation occur occasionally in severe vaginal wall prolapse

Examination is best carried out with the patient in the left lateral position using a Sims speculum.

A volsellum may be applied to the cervix so that traction will demonstrate the severity of uterine prolapse. This can cause marked discomfort and should be performed gently

Management

Prevention

1. Avoidance of perineal overstretching during labour and adequate repair thereafter
2. Encouragement to persist with postnatal pelvic floor exercises

3. Avoidance of obesity and cigarette smoking
4. Appropriate use of hormone replacement therapy in some postmenopausal women

In established cases the appropriate treatment will be determined by the following features:

1. The severity of symptoms
2. The extent of the signs — asymptomatic first degree prolapse does not require treatment
3. Age, parity and wish for further pregnancies
4. The patient's sexual activity
5. The presence of aggravating features, e.g. obesity and smoking
6. Urinary symptoms (see p. 225)
7. Other gynaecological problems, e.g. menorrhagia

Conservative treatment

1. Pelvic floor exercises will improve the tone of the pelvic floor muscles in the young parous woman but they will not produce much benefit for the woman with significant utero-vaginal prolapse
2. Ring pessaries may be used temporarily during or after pregnancy. They can be used for longer-term control in the woman who refuses or is unfit for surgery
3. The obese patient must lose weight and the smoker stop smoking. The gynaecologist cannot do his part unless the patient fulfils hers

Surgical treatment

Prolapse is not a life-threatening condition but surgery has its morbidity and occasional mortality.

1. *Anterior colporrhaphy* is appropriate for the repair of a cystocoele. It is less likely to be effective in the correction of genuine stress incontinence (see p. 225)
2. *Posterior colpoperineorrhaphy* will control a rectocoele but an enterocoele will have to be dealt with separately
3. *Manchester (Fothergill) repair* is appropriate for all degrees of prolapse in experienced hands. It combines shortening of the transverse cervical ligament with amputation of the cervix and anterior colporrhaphy. It may not deal adequately with an enterocoele.

   Surgical treatment is the best approach for the decreasing number of women with prolapse who wish to have further children.

   Full amputation of the cervix may not be necessary in less severe cases; removal of an anterior wedge of cervix may be adequate.

   Caesarean section is necessary in any subsequent pregnancy.
4. *Vaginal hysterectomy* is the ideal operation for utero-vaginal

prolapse in the presence of benign uterine pathology, as long as the uterus is not enlarged to a size greater than the equivalent of a 12 week pregnancy. It is also the operation of choice

(i) If an enterocoele is present (the utero-sacral ligaments can be used to obliterate the hernial sac)
(ii) For a procidentia, and
(iii) If the uterus is atrophic

It may also be the appropriate operation for utero-vaginal prolapse in the absence of uterine pathology, and enthusiasts claim that it is preferable to abdominal hysterectomy even in the absence of uterine descent.

SUGGESTED FURTHER READING

Tindall V R 1990 Jeffcoate's principles of gynaecology. 5th edn. Butterworths, London

Intersexes and congenital malformations of the genital tract

INTERSEX

An intersex is an individual in whom there is discordance between chromosomal, gonadal, internal genital and phenotypic sex or the sex of rearing.

This may declare itself:

1. At birth because of ambiguous external genitalia
2. During childhood because of precocious puberty
3. During adolescence because pubertal changes are inappropriate to presumed gender or because puberty fails to occur.

Some types of intersexuality may never become apparent e.g. the XYY male or XXX female.

Classification of intersexes

1. Chromosomal abnormalities
   (i) *Turner's syndrome* — see p. 172
   (ii) *Triple X female.* Some may have oligomenorrhoea and/or premature menopause but others go undetected
   (iii) *Klinefelter's syndrome* (47 XXY). Characterised by azoospermia, hypoplasia of seminiferous tubules, and perhaps gynaecomastia and eunochoidism
   (iv) *Aberration of H-Y antigen*
   XX male — maleness is due to translocation of the H-Y antigents onto an autosome or one of the X chromosomes.
   XY female — due to functional absence of H-Y. The clinical features are variable
2. Gonadal aberrations
   (i) *True hermaphrodite* — both testicular and ovarian tissue is present.
   External and internal genital sex vary widely. The commonest chromosomal structure is 46 XX
   (ii) *Gonadal agenesis* — there is no gonadal tissue but no other congenital abnormality.

The phenotype is female and the karyotype can be either 46 XX or 46 XY

(iii) *Absent anti-Mullerian factor* — noticeable at birth because of dubious genitalia. A normal vagina, uterus and tubes are present but with bilateral testes. The karyotype is 46 XY. The testis can produce androgen but not anti-Mullerian factor

3. End-organ resistance
   (i) *Testicular feminisation* — see p. 171
   (ii) *Varying degree of hypospadias* — these may be due to relative cytosol receptor deficiency

Familial or sporadic 5α-reductase deficiency will also result in the birth of children with dubious genitalia but who are genetically male. Virilisation occurs at puberty.

4. Female intersexuality due to:
   (i) Congenital adrenal hyperplasia (CAH) — the commonest cause of intersex.
   It is most frequently caused by a deficiency of 21-hydroxylase and therefore insufficient cortisol and aldosterone are produced. A female fetus will be exposed to an excess of adrenal androgens and virilisation will result.
   Profound salt loss can be life-threatening in the neonate
   (ii) Ingestion of 19-norsteroid progestogens during pregnancy; or (rarely) excess maternal androgen production. A female fetus is born virilised to a greater or lesser extent

Management

1. Check:
   Buccal smear
   Karyotype
   Urinary 17-oxosteroids
   Urinary pregnanetriol } increased in CAH
   Plasma 17α-hydroxyprogestrone
   Plasma electrolytes
2. Treat salt-losing CAH with glucocorticoids (permanently)
3. An X-ray after gastrografin instillation into the urogenital sinus will allow visualisation of the internal genitalia
4. In difficult cases assign the sex of rearing to the sex which can be made adequate for coitus

Later management

1. Any corrective surgery to the external genitalia is best carried out before the age of 3 years

2. Exploratory laparotomy is sometimes indicated but usually only in male intersexes and in true hermaphroditism
3. A male (XY) intersex showing virilism at birth will probably virilise at puberty. If the assigned sex is female the testes will need to be removed before virilisation begins at puberty
4. XY gonads should be removed in gonadal dysgenesis because of the 25% risk of malignancy
5. Testes should probably also be removed after puberty in testicular feminisation because of slightly increased risk of seminoma formation
6. If an artificial vagina is required it is best to wait until physical growth is complete
7. In gonadal agenesis or after removal of gonads oestrogens will be required to produced secondary sex characteristics at the appropriate time. Cyclical oestrogens and progestogens should be used if a uterus is present because of the risk of endometrial carcinoma if unopposed oestrogens are given over a long period of time.

CONGENITAL MALFORMATIONS OF THE GENITAL TRACT

Among the congenital anomalies which can occur are:

1. Fusion of the labia
2. Complete absence *or* duplication of the vulva (both rare)
3. Persistence of the cloaca — a serious problem. Urinary and faecal incontinence result
4. Defects of the posterior cloacal wall — faecal continence is maintained by pelvic floor muscles
5. Defects in anterior cloacal wall — affect urinary and genital tracts.

   Minor abnormalities do not cause undue problems but major defects can result in bladder exstrophy and deficient anterior abdominal wall
6. Ectopic ureter — usually an accessory ureter. The site of the orifice in relation to the bladder sphincter mechanism determines whether incontinence is present or not.

   The orifice can be difficult to locate and may not show up on excretion urography
7. Septate vagina — not uncommon and only requires division if it poses mechanical problems for coitus or childbirth. May accompany a uterine anomaly
8. Transverse vaginal membrane (including imperforate hymen). Will result in haematocolpos and cryptomenorrhoea (see p. 170)
9. Incomplete or absent vagina — both are usually associated with absence of the uterus (and possible renal tract anomalies).

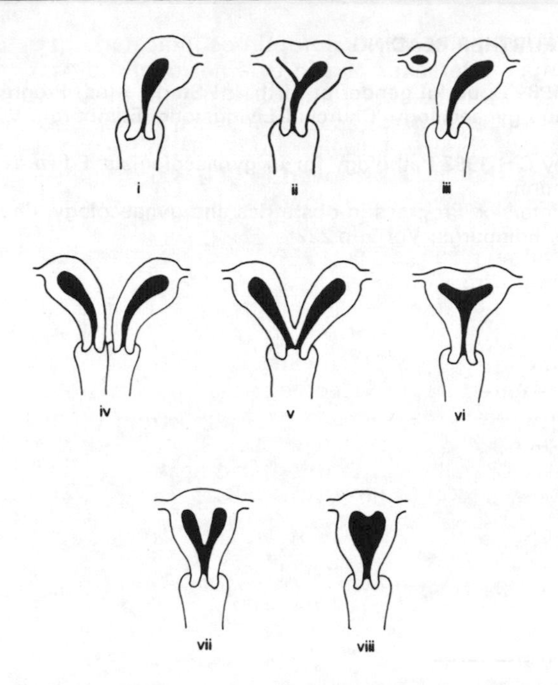

Construction of an artificial vagina may have to be considered if the vagina is non-existent. Vulvo-vaginoplasty is a relatively simple and effective procedure (see Suggested further reading)

10. Uterine anomalies.
Agenesis or arrested development of one Mullerian duct will result in one of the following
 (i) Unicornuate uterus (with tube)
 (ii) Unicornuate uterus plus some form of rudimentary horn
 (iii) The rudimentary horn may not be joined to the unicornuate uterus
Failure of, or incomplete, fusion of Mullerian duct may produce the following:
 (iv) Double uterus (didelphys) with septate vagina
 (v) Double uterus (didelphys) with normal vagina
 (vi) Arcuate deformity
 (vii) and (viii) Septate or sub-septate uterus
These anomalies may be associated with dysmenorrhoea, dyspareunia, miscarriage, pre-term labour, intrauterine growth retardation or fetal malpresentation.
 Surgical correction is only indicated for the more severe anomalies which have already produced problems.
 A uterine septum can be removed hysteroscopically.

SUGGESTED FURTHER READING

Beazley J M 1984 Doubtful gender at birth. In: Studd J (ed) Progress in obstetrics and gynaecology. Churchill Livingstone, Edinburgh, Vol 4, p 257

Fox H, Buckley C H 1982 Pathology for in gynaecologists. Edward Arnold, London

Scott J 1985 Intersex. Progress in obstetrics and gynaecology. Churchill Livingstone, Edinburgh, Vol 5, p 222

Conditions of the lower genital tract

PRURITUS VULVAE

Some local causes

1. Fungal infections — *Candida* (see p. 252), tinea cruris
2. Viral infections — herpes genitalis, genital warts, molluscum contagiosum (pox virus)
3. Parasitic infestation — scabies, pediculosis pubis, threadworms
4. Sexually transmitted infections (see pp. 99 and 215) — trichomoniasis, gonorrhoea, lymphogranuloma venereum
5. Local dermatological conditions — contact dermatitis (allergic or irritant), lichen simplex, seborrhoeic dermatitis, psoriasis etc.
6. Vulval dystrophies (see p. 244).
7. Tumours — intra-epithelial or invasive squamous cell carcinoma
8. Miscellaneous — foreign bodies, poor genital hygiene

All of these can be exacerbated by heat, moisture and friction.

Some generalised causes

1. Part of generalised dermatosis
2. Part of general medical disorder e.g. diabetes mellitus, liver disease, thyroid disease, Crohn's disease, chronic renal failure, polycythaemia, chronic lymphatic leukaemia
3. Drug reactions
4. Psychogenic causes

SWELLING OF AND AROUND THE VULVA

Among the causes are:

1. Trauma causing a haematoma
2. Infections (see above)
3. Utero-vaginal prolapse (see p. 234)
4. Cysts — sebaceous, inclusion dermoid, Wolffian duct remnants, endometriosis
5. Varicose veins

6. Enlargement of Bartholin's gland
   (i) Bartholin's adenitis — the gland is acutely painful and swollen. Abscess formation may occur. It is often due to a gonococcal infection but is not infrequently caused by staphylococci, streptococci or Gram-negative bacilli. An abscess should be incised and drained. After an infection has occurred the main duct of the gland may be blocked and a Bartholin's cyst will form. Marsupialisation rather than excision is probably the best management but not during acute infection
   (ii) Tumours — these are rare but may be benign adenomas or carcinoma (adenocarcinoma more than squamous) (see p. 247)
7. Urethral and para-urethral conditions — urethral prolapse, diverticulum or caruncle, cyst of Skene's para-urethral glands
8. Inguinal hernia or hydrocele of Canal of Nuck
9. Benign neoplasms: e.g. papilloma, fibroma, lipoma, hidradenoma (tumour of sweat glands)
10. Malignant neoplasms: primary — squamous cell carcinoma melanoma, sarcoma; secondary tumours

CHRONIC EPITHELIAL DYSTROPHIES OF THE VULVA

Vulval atrophy is normal in elderly women and is symptomless. No treatment is necessary.

The vulval dystrophies comprise a group of different conditions characterised by disorders of epithelial growth and maturation.

The characteristic symptom is pruritus. The correct diagnosis can be made only after careful consideration of the age of the patient, the appearance of the lesion, the condition of the skin elsewhere, and the histology of biopsies. Only those with abnormal and disorderly epithelial activity (cellular atypia) are sometimes pre-malignant.

Classification

Type I	Hypertrophic dystrophy	without atypia — Ia with atypia — Ib
Type II	Atrophic dystrophy (lichen sclerosus)	without atypia — IIa with atypia — IIb
Type III	Mixed dystrophy	without atypia — IIIa with atypia — IIIb

Leukoplakia, a descriptive term for irregular thickening and whitening of the vulval skin, is seen in several pathological conditions. It should not be used as a diagnostic term.

I. Hypertrophic dystrophy

Most affected women are under 50 years of age. The most

commonly affected sites are the clitoris, labia majora, interlabial sulcus, the outer surface of the labia minora and the posterior commissure. The characteristic lesions are white, red or brown plaques but appearances vary due, for example, to scratching, moisture and treatment.

Histology

(i) Hyperplasia (acanthosis) and irregular thickening of epidermis
(ii) Distorted rete ridges
(iii) Hyperkaratosis
(iv) Chronic inflammatory cell infiltrate

In 90% of cases there is no cellular atypia and, therefore, no risk of progression to neoplastic change. In the few cases with severe atypia (i.e. cellular atypia in more than two-thirds of the epithelial thickness) the risk of developing carcinoma is 10 to 25%.

II. Atrophic dystrophy (previously lichen sclerosus)

This may occur in middle age and is of unknown (possibly auto-immune) aetiology. There is an association with some other auto-immune conditions such as achlorhydria and primary biliary cirrhosis.

The commonest sites are the vulva and perianal area but extra-genital lesions may develop. It begins with irregular, flat-topped small, white papules often having a central keratotic plug.

The patches become atrophic and coalesce. The skin is paper-thin and may break down.

The introitus may shrink causing dyspareunia.

Histology

(i) Atrophic thinning of the epidermis with hyperkeratosis
(ii) Absence of dermal papillae and elastic tissue
(iii) Hyaline replacement of the collagen fibres
(iv) Lymphocytic infiltration of deep layers

III. Mixed atrophy

Areas of hyperplastic and atrophic dystrophy co-exist and each behaves as would be expected, although atypia is common in the hyperplastic areas. It comprises 10 to 15% of the vulval dystrophies.

Management of chronic epithelial dystrophies

1. Exclude deficiencies of iron, riboflavin, vitamin B12 and folic acid and achlorhydria
2. Allergies (clothing, cosmetics, toilet preparations)
3. Generalised dermatoses

4. Diabetes mellitus
5. Fungal infections

Take several widely spaced biopsies of vulval skin.

Treatment is often unsatisfactory in the absence of any underlying cause and usually entails attempted relief of pruritus and soreness.

Severe hyperkeratosis which is causing fissuring of the skin can be softened by 2% salicylic acid ointment.

Pruritus associated with hyperplastic lesions often responds to hydrocortisone cream or, if this is unsuccessful, one of the more potent topical corticosteroids (used sparingly).

Testosterone cream (2%) may be of value in atrophic lesions.

Vulvectomy should be reserved for those cases in which epithelial atypia is thought to suggest a high risk of carcinoma.

Laser therapy, cryosurgery and topical therapy with 5-fluorouracil have also been suggested.

The condition has been known to recur after vulvectomy and even skin grafting of the site.

INTRA-EPITHELIAL CARCINOMA OF THE VULVA

Atypical cells occupy the full thickness of the epithelium without any stromal invasion.

It may present as well-defined reddish-brown moist papular or plaque-like lesions accompanied by pruritus.

There may be co-existent vulval dystrophy.

Growth is slow but the lesions tend to coalesce and invasive carcinoma will supervene if the lesion is neglected.

It characteristically occurs in middle-aged to elderly women but the incidence is increasing in younger women. In up to 25% of them there is associated cervical intra-epithelial neoplasia suggesting a lower genital tract field change, possibly of viral origin.

Another rare variant is extra-mammary Paget's disease comparable to intraductal carcinoma of the breast because the apocrine sweat glands are also involved.

Management

The definitive treatment is simple vulvectomy. Paget's disease requires wide excision because recurrence is common.

A single, small, distinct and demarcated lesion can be locally excised in patients of all ages.

The factors to be considered in planning treatment are:

(i) The certainty of the diagnosis. On one hand the lesion may not in fact be neoplastic and on the other there may be areas of invasion which have been overlooked

(ii) The age of the patient and her sexual activity. The affect of complete vulvectomy on a young woman may be devastating
(iii) The size and location of the lesion
(iv) The health of the rest of the vulva e.g. the presence of infection or chronic epithelial dystrophy
(v) The ease of long-term follow up. Local excision demands follow-up

INVASIVE TUMOURS OF THE VULVA

Vulval cancer is a disease of older women. The mean age of affected women is about 60 years, and 75% of cases occur in women aged 50 years or over. It forms about 5% of all female genital tract cancers. There is an association with nulliparity and cigarette smoking.

Ninety per cent of malignant vulval neoplasms are squamous, and most develop in association with chronic vulval dystrophy or intra-epithelial neoplasia. Chronic granulomatous diseases of the vulva, e.g. syphilis, granuloma inguinale or lymphogranuloma venereum predispose to vulval cancer.

Between 15 and 30% of women with vulvar cancer have had or will develop intra-epithelial or invasive lesions of the cervix.

Presentation and spread of squamous carcinoma

An ulcer or papillary lesion may develop after a period of intractable pruritus. Continued growth is ultimately accompanied by bleeding, secondary infection and pain.

Delayed presentation is a major problem.

The commonest sites are as follows:

Labia (Labia majora three times as common as labia minora)	70%
Clitoris	15%
Perineum or fourchette	5%
Remainder	10%

Most squamous cell carcinomas of the vulva are well differentiated.

The primary route of spread is lymphatic (see below)

Spread occurs first to the superficial and deep inguinal and femoral nodes then to the external iliac and obturator nodes. The common iliac and para-aortic nodes are involved in late cases.

Contra-lateral involvement is not uncommon because of the extensive anastomosis of the lymphatic network.

Local growth progressively involves the urethra, vagina, anus and, occasionally, the bladder or rectum.

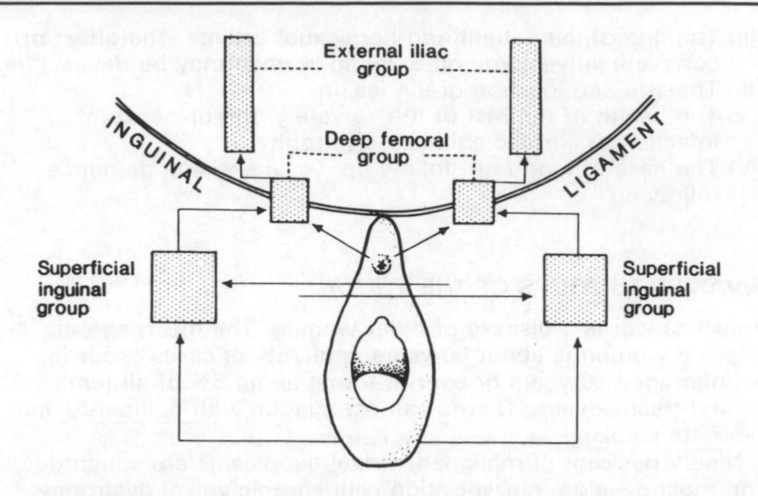

Clinical staging of squamous carcinoma

Clinical staging is unreliable: palpation of inguinal nodes is not a good guide to involvement; palpable enlarged nodes may not be affected by tumour in up to 40% of cases, and lack of enlargement may mask involvement in a similar number. Involvement of nodes is, however, an important prognostic sign, as in other malignant tumours. The 5-year survival rate in women with squamous carcinoma:

Without node involvement is about 75%
With node involvement is about 40%

Lymphangiography can be helpful in assessing pelvic node involvement.

Staging can either use a TNM (Tumour, Nodes, Metastasis) classification or clinical assessment.

TNM classification

Primary tumour (T)

- T1 Tumour confined to the vulva < 2 cm in diameter
- T2 Tumour confined to the vulva > 2 cm in diameter
- T3 Tumour of any size with adjacent spread to the urethra and/or vagina, and/or anus
- T4 Tumour of any size infiltrating the bladder (including the upper part of the urethra) mucosa, and/or the rectal mucosa and/or fixed to the bone

Regional lymph nodes (N)

- N0 No nodes palpable
- N1 Nodes palpable in either groin, not enlarged, mobile (not clinically suspicious of neoplasm)

N2 Nodes palpable in either one or both groins, enlarged, firm and mobile (clinically suspicious of neoplasm)
N3 Fixed or ulcerated nodes

Distant metastases (M)
M0 No clinical metastases
M1a Palpable deep pelvic lymph nodes
M1b Other distant metastases

Clinical stage groups
Stage I All lesions confined to the vulva, with a maximum diameter of 2 cm and no suspicious groin nodes
Stage II All lesions confined to the vulva, with a diameter > 2 cm and no suspicious groin nodes
Stage III Lesions extending beyond the vulva but without grossly positive groin nodes.
Lesions of any size confined to the vulva and having suspicious groin nodes
Stage IV Lesions with grossly positive groin nodes regardless of extent of primary
Lesions involving mucosa of rectum, bladder, urethra or involving bone
All cases with distant or palpable deep pelvic metastases

Treatment of invasive squamous cell carcinoma

Surgical treatment
The standard treatment is radical vulvectomy and bilateral lymphadenectomy (but not routinely of the pelvic nodes).
Frozen section of suspicious nodes (especially Cloquet's node) can be helpful.
Pelvic lymphadenectomy is confined to those women with extension of the lesion to urethra, clitoris, vagina or anus.
Primary closure of the wound can usually be obtained by undermining the skin flaps but tension on the suture lines at the closure junction is almost inevitable.
The major postoperative complication is wound necrosis.
The 5-year survival rate of women treated surgically is:

No node involvement	75%
Node involvement	40%

Radiotherapy
Pre-operative irradiation may reduce the size of primary lesion and make operation possible.
The normal skin of the vulva is, however, particularly susceptible to the effects of radiation, and ulceration or fibrosis are not unlikely.
Vaginal radium (or cobalt) is followed by external beam therapy. This treatment is most suitable for recurrent lesions.

When radiotherapy is carefully planned and executed, however, the results which have been reported are as follows:

Stages I and II	70% 5-year survival rate
Stages III and IV	33% 5-year survival rate

Treatment of advanced lesions is difficult and accompanied by a poor prognosis. The three possibilites are:

(i) 'Conventional' but locally more extreme surgery
(ii) Exenterative surgery
(iii) Radiotherapy combined with radical surgery

Basal cell carcinoma

Usually occurs on the labia majora beginning as a small nodule which becomes ulcerated centrally (rodent ulcer).

Lymphatics are not involved and local excision is usually adequate.

The co-existence of an invasive squamous carcinoma within the lesions must be excluded.

Melanoma

Arise from pigmented naevi containing a functional component.

Prophylactic excision of pigmented vulvar naevi is recommended because they are usually symptomless even after they have become malignant.

Treatment is by radical vulvectomy and bilateral inguinal and pelvic lymphadenectomy.

Sarcoma

This is a rare lesion and tends to occur in a younger age group than carcinoma. The mean age of patients with sarcoma is about 40 years.

Treatment is by extensive local excision but the benefit of lymphadenectomy is unclear.

Distant recurrence is common.

Bartholin's gland tumours

These are rare lesions which may be adenocarcinoma (45%), squamous carcinoma (40%), sarcoma (5%), melanoma (1%) or undifferentiated (the remainder).

Diagnosis is usually late because of the deep site of origin and the tumours may present with ulceration of the vulva and vagina.

Treatment is by extensive local excision accompanied by inguinal and pelvic lymphadenectomy.

The 5-year survival rate is probably under 10%.

VAGINAL DISCHARGE

Physiological

The vaginal fluid is a transudate through the epithelium along with desquamated cells, some polymorphs, and bacterial flora — predominantly large Gram-positive bacilli (lactobacilli).

Contributions to the fluid also comes from the cervical mucus and secretions of Skene's and Bartholin's glands. The vaginal fluid is highly acidic due to the lactic acid from the lactobacilli and glycogen from the desquamated cells.

Natural defence mechanisms of lower genital tract

1. Apposition of the labia and vaginal walls
2. Secretion of a mild fungicide by the apocrine glands of the vulva
3. Natural resistance to infection of stratified squamous epithelium (devoid of glands) of the vagina
4. Vaginal flora
5. Vaginal acidity
6. Bactericidal effects of cervical mucus

Factors affecting these defence mechanisms adversely

1. Age — infection more liable during childhood and after the menopause
2. Menstrual cycle — the alkalinity of the secretions around menses makes infection more likely
3. Pregnancy and the puerperium — a rise in pH encourages infection. Trauma at delivery with reduction in acidity by lochia and contamination with potentially pathogenic bowel flora makes the puerperium a time of particular susceptibility
4. Oestrogen-containing oral contraceptives increase the pH of vaginal fluid
5. Foreign bodies — objects such as beads or cotton wool in children or forgotten tampons in adults act as a focus for infection.
   An IUD may produce a vaginal discharge due to chronic irritation of the endometrium

The significance of a cervical ectropion

The term 'cervical erosion' should be abolished. To a patient erosion means 'ulcer', and 'ulcer' means cancer.

An ectropion is an area of columnar epithelium which has (or seems to have) extended beyond its normal boundaries. A cervical ectropion may therefore arise:

1. Congenitally — the squamo-columnar junction lies on what should be the ectocervix
2. Secondary to oestrogen-containing oral contraceptives
3. As a result of delivery — the s-c junction is normally sited but the parous cervix is patulous. (*Note*: the bivalve speculum may open the closed parous cervix and falsely give an impression of ectropion.)

Vaginal discharge may be added to by an increased secretion of mucus from a cervical ectropion.

It is not to be confused with chronic cervicitis (see p. 255).

Candida infections

Candida vaginitis and balanitis are caused by:

Candida albicans (95%)
Candida glabrato (5%)

C. albicans is not normally present in the flora of the healthy vagina.

Clinical features

1. Intense pruritus and soreness which may worsen in the evening and at night
2. Thick, white discharge (like curdled milk) adherent to the vaginal skin
3. Erythema of the vagina and labia minora which may extend peri-anally and on to the thighs

The fungus is often carried in the gastrointestinal tract and/or the mouth.

The vagina is frequently infected via the perineum but minor trauma (e.g. intercourse) facilitates infection.

Predisposing factors

1. Pregnancy — candidal vaginitis is the commonest of all infections in pregnancy. Between 15 and 20% of pregnant women may be affected
2. Menstrual cycle — growth of *Candida* is promoted at the end of the luteal phase
3. Medical disorders such as diabetes mellitus (marked increase) and iron deficiency anaemia
4. Drugs:
   (i) Oestrogen-containing oral contraceptives
   (ii) Broad-spectrum antibiotics
   (iii) Corticosteriods
   (iv) Immunosuppressive agents
5. Clothing — occlusive tights

Diagnosis

1. Clinical features — examine the vagina directly
2. Microscopy of the discharge suspended in a drop of normal saline — mycelial filaments and spores will be visible
3. Culture on glucose agar of swabs obtained in Stuart's transport medium.

Treatment

1. Fungicidal drugs e.g. nystatin or one of the imidazoles vaginally or fluconazole orally; effectiveness is > 80%

2. Genital hygiene — daily washing with bland soap and water is all that is necessary
3. Clothing — avoidance of close-fitting tights
   washing of underwear at > 80°C
4. Intercourse — no restriction necessary

Inadequate therapy is the most likely cause of chronic infections.

Note. Combined infections with *C. albicans* and *Trichomonas vaginalis* are rare due to the preferred pH of the organisms.

Trichomonal infections

These are caused by *Trichomonas vaginalis* — a flagellated protozoon.

1. Itching and/or burning sensation with dyspareunia. *Note.* Infections with *C. albicans* and *T. vaginalis* form up to 90% of pruritic vaginal discharges
2. Frothy vaginal discharge (pH 5–6) which may be white, green or brownish. The 'typical' appearance is due to gaseous fermentation by a commensal aerogenic streptococcus
3. Some vulvar oedema and congestion. Erythema is less marked than in *Candida* infections
4. The vaginal skin is reddish-purple, perhaps with dark-red spots seen best at colposcopy

They are usually sexually transmitted, and they may mask the presence (and the spread) of gonococcal infections.

The urethral and peri-urethral glands (of Skene) frequently act as a reservoir of infection.

Cervical cytology can be highly abnormal in the presence of *T. vaginalis* (see p. 257). The cervical smear must be repeated after adequate treatment of the infection.

Diagnosis

1. Clinical features — examine the vagina directly; the vaginal pH is alkaline (pH 5–6)
2. Microscopy of the discharge suspended in a drop of normal saline — motile flagellated protozoa are seen (about the same size as a polymorph leukocyte)
3. Culture of swabs collected in Bushby's brown transport medium

Treatment

Metronidazole for both partners.

Gonococcal infections (see also p. 215)

These are due to *Neisseria gonorrhoeae*. This bacterium attacks columnar and transitional epithelium e.g. in the urethra, para-urethral ducts and glands, endocervix and anorectal canal.

Clinical features
Painful swelling of the vulva
Dysuria and frequency due to urethritis
Orifices of urethral, para-urethral and Bartholin's glands are congested
Greenish vaginal discharge 2–7 days (or longer) after intercourse with infected partner
Vaginal skin red and oedematous
Purulent exudate from the urethra and cervix
Salpingo-oophoritis may develop (see p. 214)

Diagnosis
1. Clinical features and history of contact
2. Gram staining of purulent exudates — *N. gonorrhoeae* are Gram-negative intra- and extracellular diplococci (i.e. they appear in pairs)
3. Swabs from potentially infected sites. The full range for accurate sampling is endocervix, urethra, rectum and throat.
   High vaginal swabs are of no value in most cases
4. Culture by direct inoculation on modified Thayer–Martin plates. Swabs can be transported to the laboratory in Stuart's transport medium

Treatment
1. *Penicillin-sensitive organisms*: probenecid 1 to 2 g orally then procaine penicillin 2.4 to 4.8 mega-units intramuscularly, *or*
   probenecid + ampicillin 3 g orally
2. β-Lactamase-producing-penicillin-resistant organisms: use erythromycin or spectinomycin. The combination of the β-lactamase inhibitor, clavulanic acid and amoxycillin can be helpful in this context
3. *Patients allergic to penicillin*: use erythromycin or spectinomycin

Contacts must be followed up.

Infections with other organisms
1. *Gardnerella vaginalis* may cause discharge on its own or in combination with anaerobic organisms. It is also found in over 20% of healthy, symptomless women
2. All pyogenic organisms can become pathogenic after trauma, in the presence of a foreign body, or after delivery. Such organisms include:
   Staphylococci
   Streptococci

Gram-negative bacilli
Anaerobes

They are usually saprophytic in the vagina

3. Vulvo-vaginitis may arise due to infestation with amoebae, schistosomes, or threadworms

BENIGN CONDITIONS OF THE VAGINA AND CERVIX

1. Gaertner duct cyst

These arise from of the mesonephric (Wolffian) duct and therefore occur antero-laterally in the vagina. They may be single or multiple and of varied size. Histology shows a single layer of cuboidal epithelium. Treatment is by excision or marsupialisation.

2. Vaginal inclusion cysts

Usually small and often multiple resulting from inversion of small fragments of vaginal skin after delivery or vaginal surgery.

3. Endometriosis (see p. 183)

4. Condylomata acuminata

Genital warts are caused by Papova (DNA) virus. They are sexually transmitted and therefore may be accompanied by other STDs. They grow larger in pregnancy and tend to regress after delivery.

Treatment is by podophyllin, saturated trichloracetic acid or electrocautery. Severe cases can be destroyed by laser (under GA).

5. Papillomas of vagina and cervix

Cervical papillomas are more common than vaginal ones. Clinically they can be difficult to differentiate from genital warts. They derive from the squamous epithelium with various degrees of keratinisation. The stalk is of fibrous connective tissue. They need to be removed surgically and sent for histological examination because they have a significant malignant potential.

6. Other (rare) benign tumours — e.g. fibroleiomyoma

7. Chronic cervicitis

This is characterised by a hypertrophied, spongy cervix, in parous women presenting with seemingly purulent vaginal discharge.

An ectropion (p. 251) may be present and/or several small or large retention cysts of the cervical mucous glands (Nabothian follicles).

If treatment is necessary it can be carried out in outpatients using cryocautery.

8. Cervical polyp

This is a smooth, pedunculated growth from the columnar epithelium of the endocervix. Polyps can be due to hypertrophy of the mucous membrane or may be true benign neoplasms.

It is the commonest lesion of the cervix.

Size varies from a few millimetres up to 2 cm in diameter.

The surface epithelium of the polyp is often ulcerated causing the intermenstrual bleeding with which they most commonly present.

Cervical polyps are of low malignant potential but rarely a seemingly innocent polyp is the early lesion of sarcoma botryoides. They can be avulsed by twisting and, if necessary, the base can be cauterised. Histological examination should also be carried out.

9. Squamous metaplasia of the cervix

This is a focal or diffuse replacement of the glandular epithelium by squamous cells. The process probably arises from reserve or basal cells in the original epithelium. The pattern and form of the cells may be confused with carcinoma-in-situ (see below).

INTRA-EPITHELIAL NEOPLASIA OF THE VAGINA AND CERVIX

Nomenclature and definitions

Dyskaryosis — a cytological term which refers to abnormalities of individual cells such as enlargement and hyperchromasia of the nuclei with uneven chromatin distribution, irregular nuclear membrane and multinucleation.

Dysplasia — a histological diagnosis which describes abnormalities of epithelium. It has been defined by WHO as a lesion in which part of the thickness of the epithelium is replaced by cells showing varying degrees of atypia.

Carcinoma-in-situ refers to lesions in which all or most of the epithelium shows the following features:

1. Loss of stratification and polarity throughout the full thickness of the epithelium
2. Variation in size and shape of cells
3. Increased nuclear/cytoplasmic ratio
4. Frequent bizarre mitoses
5. The basement membrane is intact

The only difference between dysplasia and carcinoma-in-situ is one of degree.

CERVICAL INTRA-EPITHELIAL NEOPLASIA — CIN

This is a general term which includes all the above abnormalities.

Cytology	*Grade*	*Histology*
Mild dyskaryosis	1	Mild dysplasia
Moderate dyskaryosis	2	Moderate dysplasia
Severe dyskaryosis	3	Severe dysplasia and carcinoma-in-situ

Cytological characteristics of CIN

CIN 1: *Superficial cell* (*mild*) — nuclear abnormalities with abundant cytoplasm and angular cell borders

CIN 2: *Intermediate cell* (*moderate*) — nucleus much larger in proportion to the whole cell than normally but occupying less than 50% of the cell

CIN 3: *Parabasal cell* (*severe*) — the nucleus occupies more than 50% of the cell. The cell border is round or oval

The cytology report emphasises the most immature cells present.

Histological characteristics of CIN grades

CIN 1 (mild dysplasia)
- (i) Upper two-thirds of epithelium exhibits relatively good differentiation
- (ii) Mild nuclear abnormality, most marked in basal layer
- (iii) Few mitotic figures confined to basal third

CIN 2 (moderate dysplasia)
- (i) Upper half of epithelium is well differentiated
- (ii) Moderate nuclear abnormalities
- (iii) Mitotic figures (some abnormal) present in basal two-thirds

CIN 3
- (i) Maturation confined to superficial one-third of epithelium or absent
- (ii) Nuclear abnormalities marked and throughout full thickness
- (iii) Mitotic figures may be numerous, at all levels and with many abnormal configurations

Aetiology

The cause of CIN and cervical cancer have the same origin. Approximately 30–50% of cases of CIN will, if left untreated, progress to invasive disease.

Epidemiology

CIN and cervical cancer are sexually transmitted diseases. The disease is extremely rare in nuns, and relatively common in prostitutes. Associated characteristics of affected women include number of sexual partners, divorce, venereal disease and religious or cultural factors: for example, the relative immunity of Jewesses is likely to be due to religious codes of practice. *The common denominator appears to be age at first intercourse.*

A male factor is also involved. The wives of men with prostatic or penile cancer have a higher risk of cervical cancer than have the wives of those whose first partners died of cervical cancer.

Cervical neoplasia is most common among lower socio-economic groups. Prolonged use of oral contraception and cigarette smoking are associated with an increased risk of cervical neoplasia.

The age specific prevalence for CIN 1 and CIN 2 is 20 to 29 years, and for CIN 3 it is 36–39 years.

Biology

The transformation zone (TZ) is a circumferential region of tissue between the vaginal (squamous) and endocervical (columnar) tissue. It is composed of columnar epithelium which has descended on to the ectocervix, although the final border between the columnar and squamous epithelium is usually not finally defined until adult life. The columnar epithelium of the TZ metaplases to a varying degree to squamous epithelium. This process exposes the epithelium to neoplastic transformation. The precise mutagen involved is uncertain. Two groups of viruses have come under the closest scrutiny — herpes genitalis and human papillomovirus (HPV), the latter currently being the most-favoured candidate. HPV cannot be cultured but may be typed by DNA in situ hybridisation techniques. HPV type 16 has been found in over 90% of invasive cervical cancer, but it is uncommonly found in condyloma acuminata. The reverse is true for HPV types 6 and 11.

Cytological screening and the prevention of cervical cancer

The success of cytological screening programmes depends on the percentage of women at risk screened. Comprehensive programmes have achieved significant reductions in both the incidence of, and death rate from, the disease. In British Columbia, for example, the prevalence has been reduced seven-fold. The remaining unscreened women at risk have a much greater risk of having (and dying from) the disease.

The number of women screened and the frequency of screening depends on the resources available. One recommended screening policy is as follows:

1. The first smear should be taken at 25 years of age in women attending family planning, antenatal and venereal disease clinics
2. In the remainder of the sexually active population smears should commence at 30 years of age

3. The first smear should be repeated a year later (in case the first was falsely negative)
4. Thereafter intervals of 3 to 5 years are adequate
5. Regular testing can probably stop from 70 years of age if previous smears have been normal

Current cytological screening practice in the UK has not reduced the mortality rate from cervical cancer; therefore greater emphasis should be placed on screening women who have never had a smear rather than increasing the frequency of screening women who have.

Although the majority of invasive cervical cancers occur in women over the age of 35 years, the incidence of the disease is increasing in women under 35 (see p. 263). The disease in this group seems to be more aggressive than in most older women. It is likely that there are least two different types of cervical cancer whose 'life cycles' have considerably different time courses.

A screening policy which does not screen women before the age of 35 is unacceptable because it will fail to detect increasingly common pre-malignant change (and therefore curable disease) in younger women.

Cervical smears

The proper taking, interpretation and follow-up of cervical smears are fundamental to the whole screening programme.

Specimens for cervical and/or vaginal cytology are usually taken with a wooden (or plastic) Ayre spatula.

The days of menstrual loss are best avoided.

The slide must not be allowed to dry in air because the cells become distorted.

Fixation is in alcohol and ether or with a wax-based resin. All smears must be accompanied by adequate information about the patient.

False-negative smears are those reported as normal in a patient who has a neoplastic lesion of the cervix. This may be due to:

1. An error in taking the smear — cervix not properly sampled
2. Technical problem — smear too thin, too thick, too bloody, poorly fixed or poorly stained
3. Diagnostic failures — misinterpretation by the cytologist
4. The size of the lesion (too small) so that very few cells exfoliate

The reported frequency of false-negative smears is between 1.8 and 20%!

False-positive smears are those in which malignant changes are seen but subsequent full examination of the cervix fails to reveal them. They may be due to errors in the laboratory, therefore positive smears should be repeated before any surgery is contemplated. However, the cytologist may be correct and the source of the malignant cells may have remained undetected higher in the cervical canal and than detected at colposcopy or even cone biopsy.

Evaluation of the patient with CIN

In the majority of patients with CIN the cervix will look quite normal to the naked eye.

No patient with cytological evidence of CIN should be treated without prior colposcopic assessment.

Colposcopy

Among the indications for colposcopy in primary diagnosis are abnormal cytology and suspicious vaginal or cervical lesions even if cytology is negative. The aims of colposcopic examination of the cervix in women with CIN are:

1. To demarcate the boundaries of the transformation zone (TZ)
2. To rule out invasive disease by directed biopsies
3. To confirm/refute the suspicion raised by cytology
4. To plan appropriate treatment

Treatment of CIN

Intra-epithelial neoplasia is a localised problem and can be treated satisfactorily by destruction of the abnormal epithelium.

The method used is less important than the assurance that all neoplastic tissue is destroyed or removed. Among the suggested methods of treatment are:

Cone biopsy

This can provide both firm diagnosis and comprehensive treatment. It is even more effective if colposcopically directed (99% primary cure rate). The operation is not without immediate or longer-term hazard such as:

(i) Primary or secondary haemorrhage
(ii) Local infection
(iii) Cervical stenosis (small cones)
(iv) Cervical incompetence (large cones)

Fertility is probably unaffected, but mid-trimester abortion and pre-term delivery may be more common and this seems to be directly related to the size of the cone removed.

If the raw area of the cervix is covered by mobilising the remainder of the cervical epithelium residual CIN in the endocervical crypts may be covered and remain occult.

Incomplete excision by the conisation requires further definitive surgery (e.g. another cone biopsy, or hysterectomy) in the not-too-distant future.

Loop diathermy excision of TZ

This can often be carried out as an out-patient. A major benefit

= Large loop excision of TZ
(LLETZ)

over destructure methods discussed below is that the area removed is available for histology.

Local destruction of the whole TZ

This can be achieved by carbon dioxide laser, cold coagulation, cryocautery, radical electrocoagulation diathermy, or electrocautery. These have the advantage that they are not associated with significant morbidity (including fertility-related problems). In addition, laser, cryocautery and cold coagulation may be performed as outpatient procedures with or without local anaesthesia.

Before selecting a patient for a local destructive technique or diathermy excision the patient must be assessed by a competent colposcopist who:

(i) Is able to see the lesion and the transformation zone in its entirety
(ii) Is certain that there is no evidence of invasion by taking colposcopically directed biopsies
(iii) Is certain that there is no suspicion (cytologically or colposcopically) of abnormal columnar cells suggesting an endometrial neoplasm
(iv) Is assured that there will be regular cytological and colposcopic follow-up

Hysterectomy

This may be the method of choice for CIN 3 in women who have completed their family, who wish complete assurance of cure, and/or in whom follow-up is likely to be difficult.

Removal of a cuff of vagina is not necessary.

Cervical human papilloma virus (HPV) infection

Genital tract infections with HPV are increasingly common, as is the association with CIN and invasive disease. The *papillary condyloma acuminatum* is the commonest but the condylomas are, rarely, inverted. Non-condylomatous wart virus infections are being recognised more commonly.

The classical cytological and histological feature of HPV infection is koilocytosis, i.e. infected cells have an irregular and hyperchromatic nucleus with a halo around them and margination of the cytoplasm.

HPV infection may be found adjacent to CIN or in association with it, in the same area of epithelium. Treatment should be as is appropriate for the observed degree of CIN.

VAGINAL INTRA-EPITHELIAL NEOPLASIA (VAIN)

VAIN is asymptomatic and detected only by cytological and/or colposcopic examination. Its appearances are as for CIN. The treatment options for VAIN are:

1. Laser vaporisation
2. Intravaginal 5-fluorouracil
3. Radiation
4. Surgical excision

If a hysterectomy is being performed in the presence of CIN all the affected epithelium must be excised with the hysterectomy specimen. (In approximately 4% of women it extends on to the vaginal walls.)

When detected following hysterectomy management is difficult, because the angles of the vagina are difficult to assess by cytology and colposcopy.

CARCINOMA OF THE VAGINA

Primary malignant tumours of the vagina are rare, and an invasive lesion is more likely to be due to secondary spread.

Squamous cell carcinoma

This is the commonest histological type and accounts for 1–2% of all gynaecological malignancies. Most occur between the ages of 55 and 70 years with a peak incidence of about 65 years. The commonest presenting symptoms are vaginal discharge, and bleeding as a result of ulceration of the tumour. The most frequent site is the posterior vaginal wall.

Staging

Stage 0:	Intra-epithelial carcinoma
Stage I:	Limited to vaginal wall
Stage II:	Outside the vagina but not to pelvic side walls
Stage III:	To the pelvic side walls and/or symphysis pubis
Stage IV:	Extension beyond the true pelvis or involving the bladder or rectum

The lesions are usually moderately undifferentiated.

Tumours in the lower third of the vagina spread to the inguinal nodes like carcinoma of the vulva (p. 248).

In the upper vagina, spread is similar to that of carcinoma of the cervix (p. 264).

Treatment

Radiotherapy is the treatment of choice except if the lesion is at the introitus, when radical surgery may be possible. Five-year survival rates are:

Stage I:	85%
Stage II:	55%
Stage III:	30%
Stage IV:	<10%

Adenocarcinoma

This rare tumour is most often found in young women with a history of intra-uterine exposure to diethyl stilboestrol (DES). There is therefore also an association with vaginal adenosis.

Some lesions have been detected merely by screening young women whose mothers took DES during pregnancy. In the others abnormal vaginal bleeding or discharge are the commonest presenting symptoms.

Routine vaginal cytology is unreliable.

The most frequent histological type is a clear cell adenocarcinoma, and the commonest site is the upper third of the vagina. Spread is by local extension and by the lymphatics and bloodstream.

Staging

As for squamous carcinoma of the cervix.

Treatment

Radical hysterectomy, vaginectomy and pelvic lymphadenectomy is preferred. Radiotherapy can be used if expert surgery is not available, or in young women with small lesions (because the remainder of the vagina, adjacent structures and ovarian function can be preserved). Five-year survival rates are:

Stage I:	80%
Stage II:	< 20%
Stages III and IV:	None

Secondary vaginal tumours

Metastatic carcinoma of the vagina is commoner than a primary cancer. It occurs frequently in carcinoma of the cervix, sometimes after carcinoma of the endometrium and occasionally in carcinoma of the ovary or choriocarcinoma. It may rarely follow hypernephroma or carcinoma of the colon or rectum.

CARCINOMA OF THE CERVIX

Cervical cancer is second to ovarian as the commonest malignant tumour of the genital tract, comprising 30% of the total.

Despite an overall fall in incidence, particularly among older women, the peak age is still 50 to 59 years. However, in the past decade the incidence has doubled in women under 40 years. The mortality has almost trebled in women under 34 years of age.

It is more common in multiparous women than nulliparous women. Women who have had multiple sexual partners are at particular risk (for further consideration see p. 257). The condition is more common in women from the lower socio-economic groups. Women of Jewish origin are relatively immune to cancer of the cervix.

Ninety-five per cent of the tumours are squamous and the remainder adenocarcinoma.

Squamous carcinoma

Histology

Cell characteristics

(i) Loss of stratification
(ii) Various degrees of immaturity and lack of differentiation
(iii) Pleomorphism of cells and nuclei
(iv) Hyperchromatic nuclei
(v) Abundant and atypical mitoses
(vi) Giant cell formation

Architecture

(i) The malignant epithelium has broken through the basement membrane
(ii) The stroma is penetrated by more than 3 mm (see Clinical staging)
(iii) Lymphocyte and polymorph infiltration of stroma

The more immature and undifferentiated the tumour the more malignant it is (and more radiosensitive).

Spread

Early spread occurs by local infiltration.

Upward spread into the body of the uterus is uncommon, and forward spread into the bladder occurs late. Obstruction of the ureters is common (many deaths occur due to uraemia).

Lymphatic spread first involves a primary group of nodes:

Parametrial	Hypogastric
Vesico-vaginal	Obturator
Recto-vaginal	External iliac

and then a secondary group of nodes:

Sacral	Vaginal (deep and superficial)
Common iliac	Para-aortic

Even in clinically assessed stage Ib disease pelvic lymph nodes will be affected in about 15% of patients.

Clinical features

It may be asymptomatic (even to a late stage) and be detected by routine cervical smear or examination.

Once it is clinically detectable, intermenstrual, postmenopausal or postcoital bleeding are the commonest presenting symptoms.

Vaginal discharge is less frequent and a later development. Pain occurs only in the very late stages.

On examination the cervix may:

1. Appear normal (e.g. intra-epithelial or endocervical)

2. Be hard with a granular 'erosion' which bleeds to touch
3. Be ulcerated

Moderately advanced growths may be exophytic (polypoid), infiltrative or ulcerative.

Management

1. Check full blood count, urea, and electrolytes
2. Carry out chest X-ray and excretion urography (IVP) (a bone survey for metastasis is not routine).
   The value of lymphangiography remains controversial. Close co-operation between gynaecologist and radiotherapist is vital
3. Carry out pelvic examination (vaginal and rectal) under anaesthesia to assess the extent of the disease. This is the definitive staging on which the success of treatment is assessed.
4. Proceed to:
   (i) Dilatation and fractional curettage of the uterus
   (ii) Cervical biopsy for histology
   (iii) Cystoscopy — looking for bullous oedema which suggests involvement of the underlying muscle. (The first insertion of caesium can be carried out at this time if need be.)

Clinical staging

Stage 0:	Intra-epithelial carcinoma (p. 257)
Stage I:	Invasive carcinoma confined to the cervix
Stage Ia:	No lesion visible at clinical examination, and stromal invasion is less than 3 mm (micro-invasion)
Stage Ib:	All other stage I lesions
Stage II:	The carcinoma extends beyond the cervix but not to the pelvic side wall; and/or the upper two-thirds of the vagina are involved
Stage IIa:	No parametrial involvement
Stage IIb:	Obvious parametrial involvement
Stage III:	The carcinoma extends to the pelvic side wall and/or the lower one-third of the vagina is involved. Presence of hydronephrosis or non-functioning kidney
Stage IIIa:	No extension to the pelvic wall
Stage IIIb:	Extension to the pelvic wall
Stage IV:	The carcinoma extends beyond the true pelvis or involves the bladder or rectum (bullous oedema is excluded)

Treatment of stage Ia (micro-invasive) carcinoma

The definition and management of micro-invasion are still hotly debated and consensus is not possible from the available literature (see Suggested further reading).

Working definition
A micro-invasive lesion is one in which the carcinoma invades the stroma in one or more places to a depth of 3 mm or less below the basement membrane and in which lymphatics and blood vessels cannot be seen to be involved. The following qualifications are necessary:

1. It is not possible to examine the whole specimen histologically in every case
2. It is difficult to distinguish extensive gland or cleft involvement from stromal invasion
3. If clumps of tumour cells can be seen in vascular spaces, even if invasion is minimal, lymph nodes are involved in up to 25% of cases

Treatment

1. Conservative therapy as for stage 0 (see p. 260) can be considered when invasion is minimal in young women who are anxious to retain fertility. Close cytological and colposcopic follow-up is necessary
2. Simple hysterectomy should be used:
   (i) For older women or in those whose family is complete
   (ii) When the pathologist is uncertain of the diagnosis of micro-invasion

   A cuff of vagina should be taken if the transformation zone extends on to the vagina.
3. Radical therapy (as for stage Ib) is probably best for those with clumps of tumour cells in vascular spaces, and certainly if stromal invasion is more than 3 mm (macro-invasion)

   The cure rate should be close to 100%.

Treatment of stage Ib and IIa
The choice is between radical (Wertheim's) hysterectomy and radiotherapy.

Radical hysterectomy
The lesion most suitable for treatment by radical hysterectomy is one which is confined to the cervix or with only minimal extension beyond it, particularly in the younger patient. The procedure involves removal of the uterus, cervix, parametria, upper one-third to one-half of the vagina and as many pelvic lymph nodes as possible.

It is now thought unnecessary to sacrifice ovaries, and this is a great advantage, particularly in younger women.

Advantages of surgery

1. The cervix and uterus are excised and no recurrence of tumour is then possible
2. Treatment is less prolonged
3. The ovaries need not be removed in young patients with early disease
4. Early and late complications of radiotherapy are avoided
5. Infection is no bar to treatment (unlike radiotherapy)
6. Potential radio-resistance is overcome
7. The prognostic information obtained is more use

Disadvantages of surgery

1. Only selected patients benefit from it
2. It is more hazardous than radiotherapy
3. Bladder dysfunction is common
4. The vagina is shortened

Complications of surgery
Immediate and short-term: e.g. anaesthetic problems, haemorrhage, shock, sepsis, thrombo-embolism.

Long-term: e.g. ureteric and rectal fistulae; lymphocyst — a collection of lymph on the pelvic side wall; urinary retention.

Radiotherapy
The tumour itself and any paracervical spread are attacked using intrauterine and intravaginal caesium 137.

The pelvic lymph nodes and their lymphatics are dealt with mainly by external irradiation.

The aim is to deliver 6000–7500 roentgens (R) at point A (2 cm lateral to the midline; 2 cm above the lateral fornix in the same sagittal plane as the uterus). Point B (5 cm from the midline at the same level and the same place) receives only 25% of the dosage according to the inverse square law.

External irradiation (preferably by linear accelerator) should deliver 5000–7500 R to the pelvic side walls.

There is considerable variation in individual policies and regimes but the overall aims are the same.

Complications of radiotherapy

1. *Vaginal stenosis* may develop in up to 85% of irradiation patients.

   This falls to 30% if topical (i.e. vaginal) oestrogen therapy is used from completion of therapy. No cytological abnormalities have been reported associated with topical oestrogen therapy and the tumour is not oestrogen-dependent
2. *Urinary tract injuries* may occur. Some frequency and dysuria is inevitable. Bladder ulcers can be difficult to cure.

Vesico-vaginal fistulae occur rarely and usually some 3–8 months after treatment.

Uretero-vaginal fistulae are more liable to occur when radiotherapy and surgery are combined

3. *Intestinal complications* may arise, varying from diarrhoea to rectal fistulae

Combined radiotherapy and surgery

Three caesium insertions can be carried out on days 0, 7 and 21. A Wertheim's radical hysterectomy is undertaken 4–6 weeks later. If lateral pelvic wall nodes are affected supplementary external radiation is required.

Note: if invasive carcinoma is diagnosed as a result of cone biopsy definitive treatment should be deferred for 6 weeks, if possible, to allow healing to occur. Otherwise the complications of radiotherapy and/or surgery are increased.

Results of treatment

Whatever the method used to treat carcinoma of the cervix, the 5-year survival rates are comparable at:

Stage Ib: 85–90%
Stage IIa: 70–75%

(If lymph nodes are positive, survival drops to 50–60%.)

The results of surgery improve and its complications lessen with the expertise of the surgeon. To ensure the best treatment for each patient the following criteria must be met.

1. There must be close co-operation between the surgical and radiotherapeutic teams
2. Any surgery should be carried out by, or under the guidance of, a gynaecologist adequately trained in radical surgery and able to cope with any contingency
3. Close follow-up must be organised

Treatment of carcinoma of the cervix — stages IIb to IV

The treatment of choice is radiotherapy.

Pelvic exenteration is applicable when radiotherapy is unlikely to be effective or when the tumour has not regressed during radiotherapy.

Anterior exenteration — bladder removed in conjunction with radical hysterectomy and lymphadenectomy.

Posterior exenteration — rectum removed.

Total exenteration — both bladder and rectum removed. These operations are justified only if there is some expectation of useful life as a result. They are not applicable if extra-pelvic metastases are present. A terminal colostomy and ileal conduit are to be preferred to a 'wet' colostomy. Five-year survival rates are as follows:

Stage IIb 50–60%

(LN) pretreatment surgical staging / transperitoneal — retroperitoneal
→ LN resection if involved
→ ↑ cure

Stage III: 30–35%
Stage IV: < 10%

Recurrent carcinoma of the cervix

If the tumour recurs it usually does so within 18 months of treatment. The main sites are:

Deep pelvis:	35%
Distant spread:	30%
Lateral pelvis:	15%
Bladder or rectum:	10%
Central pelvis:	10%

The most frequent signs and symptoms are:
Renewed vaginal bleeding
Pain
Weight loss
Evidence of urinary tract obstruction

If radiotherapy has not been used, or was incomplete, then further treatment is possible.

Occasionally exenteration can be carried out.

Palliation is usually all that can be offered.

For relief of pain in advanced cancer see p. 223.

The ultimate causes of death, in order of frequency, are uraemia, cachexia, severe haemorrhage, complications of treatment and, rarely, remote metastases to vital organs.

Adenocarcinoma of the cervix

These tumours are rare but they tend to grow and spread as squamous carcinoma. They respond equally to radiotherapy or surgery.

Treatment is as for squamous carcinoma.

SUGGESTED FURTHER READING

Cartier R 1985 Practical colposcopy, 2nd edn. Laboratoire Cartier, Paris

Delgado G 1983 Cancer of the vulva. In: Studd J (ed) Progress in obstetrics and gynaecology. Churchill Livingstone, Edinburgh, Vol 3, p. 187

Fox H (ed) 1984 Gynaecological pathology: advances, perspectives and problems. Clinics in obstetrics and gynaecology. Saunders, London, Vol 11, No. 1

Kenney A 1985 Carcinoma of the vulva — which operation when? In: Studd J (ed) Progress in obstetrics and gynaecology. Churchill Livingstone, Edinburgh, Vol 5, p. 390

Shepherd J J, Monaghan J M 1985 Clinical gynaecological oncology. Blackwell, Oxford

Singer A 1985 Cancer of the cervix: diagnosis and treatment. Clinics in obstetrics and gynaecology. Saunders, London, Vol 12, No. 1

Tindall V R 1990 Jeffcoate's principles of gynaecology. 5th edn. Butterworth, London

Conditions of the body of the uterus and Fallopian tubes

ENDOMETRIAL POLYP (ADENOMA)

These polyps are usually multiple before the menopause and may be a component of endometrial hyperplasia. After the menopause they are usually single (or few in number). They tend to recur. Most are symptomless but they may be associated with:

Menorrhagia
Intermenstrual bleeding
Postcoital bleeding
Postmenopausal bleeding

They are easily removed by small ovum forceps and curettage.

Hysteroscopy may be of value also because a polyp may elude curettage.

All polyps should be sent for histology to exclude malignant change.

UTERINE FIBROIDS

A leiomyoma is a well circumscribed benign uterine tumour derived mainly from smooth muscle but containing some fibrous connective tissue elements. It is the commonest tumour of the female genital tract, being present in at least 20% of women over the age of 35. The peak age incidence of symptoms is between 35 and 45 years.

In Caucasian, but not black, women they are associated with nulliparity or relative infertility.

Growth may be related to oestrogen stimulation.

Sites of origin

Intramural — within uterine wall
Subserous — projecting from the peritoneal surface of the uterus
Intraligamentary — between the layers of the broad ligament
Submucous — indenting the uterine cavity
Cervical

Submucous fibroids may become polypoidal and subserous ones pedunculated. Pedunculated fibroids may lose their uterine attachment and gain a secondary blood supply (parasitic fibroid).

Gross characteristics
They may be small, medium-sized or large, and are usually multiple. They are usually firm, but can be soft and cystic if degeneration has taken place.

They are white and characteristically whorled in appearance.

There is a false capsule of compressed uterine muscle which allows easy enucleation (cf. adenomyosis).

Histology
Groups and bundles of smooth muscle fibres are interlaced in twists and whorls. The fibrous component becomes more marked as the tumour enlarges.

Clinical features
1. The majority are symptomless
2. Increased menstrual loss is usually caused by submucous fibroids. Intermenstrual bleeding may be due to a fibroid polyp with an ulcerated tip. (*Note*: Atypical menstrual symptoms may be due to a concurrent but separate pathology.)
3. Pressure effects may give rise to bladder symptoms and interfere with venous return
4. Abdominal swelling may be noted
5. Pain is not a common symptom unless the fibroid has become complicated (see below)
6. There is a rare association with polycythaemia

Differential diagnosis must include all causes of pelvic swellings. It is not always easy to discern clinically between a solid ovarian tumour and a pedunculated fibroid. The difference between a fibroid and an adenomyoma may not be apparent until surgical removal is attempted.

Potential effects of fibroids on pregnancy
Subfertility
Abortion and pre-term labour
Malpresentations
Obstructed labour (rare)
Third stage problems
Delayed involution postpartum

Complications of fibroids
1. Torsion of pedicle
2. Haemorrhage

3. Infection — usually at the tip of a fibroid polyp
4. Hyaline degeneration — present to some degree in most moderate to large-sized fibroids. The tumour may be painful, enlarged and soft. Cystic degeneration follows
5. Red degeneration (necrobiosis) — occurs typically during pregnancy and is due to infarction of the centre of the tumour during mid-pregnancy. Characteristically the fibroid suddenly enlarges and is painful and tender. It can be mistaken for placental abruption or any acute abdominal emergency. It is treated conservatively during pregnancy
6. Calcification — usually seen postmenopausally and/or in pedunculated fibroids
7. Malignant change occurs in under 0.5% of cases. The fibroid may grow suddenly and be painful and tender. It is difficult to differentiate clinically from other degenerative changes

On removal, the centre of the fibroid is soft and homogeneous. The histology shows a leiomyosarcoma (see p. 275).

Treatment

Conservative management is appropriate:
When the tumours are small, the diagnosis is certain and there are no symptoms
During pregnancy
Near the menopause when there are no symptoms and the tumour is not enlarging

LHRH analogues can be used in the short term to reduce the size of fibroids in:
Women approaching the menopause
Those with contra-indications to surgery
As an adjunct to surgery if fibroids are large.
Further studies of their use are necessary.

Surgery is indicated if:
The fibroids are causing symptoms or are growing rapidly
They are larger than a size corresponding to a 16-week pregnancy
The diagnosis is in doubt
They are likely to complicate a future pregnancy
Hysterectomy is the definitive treatment. Myomectomy is indicated for those women who are subfertile, want more children or refuse to undergo hysterectomy.

It may be possible to resect small submucous fibroids endoscopically.

Rupture of a myomectomy scar during subsequent pregnancy or labour is very rare, and vaginal delivery is often possible. (Any fibroids found at Caesarean section should usually be left undisturbed.)

ENDOMETRIAL CARCINOMA

This tumour comprises 25 to 30% of all gynaecological malignancies. The incidence is low before 40 years of age, rises sharply until 55 years and then falls slightly.

A greater proportion of women with endometrial carcinoma are postmenopausal than is the case in carcinoma of the cervix.

Nulliparous women are 2 to 3 times more likely to develop it than are paraous women, although half the women with the disease will have had one or more pregnancies.

There is no relationship with social class.

There is an association with gross obesity, polycystic ovary syndrome, and possibly diabetes mellitus.

Role of hormone replacement therapy (HRT)

There is an increased risk of endometrial cancer when unopposed oestrogen replacement is given after the climacteric.

If HRT is necessary in a patient who still has her uterus it should be given cyclically combined with progestogen for the last 7 to 13 days of the cycle.

Outpatient endometrial sampling should be carried out if unopposed oestrogens have been taken for more than 6 months.

Irregular vaginal bleeding is an indication for urgent curettage.

Pathology

It is nearly always adenocarcinoma, but there may be squamous elements (adenoacanthoma).

It may be diffuse or circumscribed.

Histology

In most cases the diagnosis is clear-cut due to the disordered architecture, atypical glands, and abnormal activity and characteristics of the cells.

Atypical proliferative varieties of hyperplasia may be difficult to distinguish from adenocarcinoma.

Benign cystic glandular hyperplasia is not liable to become malignant, but atypical hyperplasia is, and removal of the uterus is recommended.

Spread is direct within the endometrium and, to a lesser degree, into the myometrium.

Penetration to the serosa is uncommon.

Lymphatic spread is mainly along the ovarian vessels to the para-aortic nodes.

Pelvic lymph node involvement is not common except when the tumour has spread to the cervix or there is marked invasion of the myometrium.

Clinical features

Irregular vaginal bleeding — intermenstrual or postmenopausal. Watery vaginal discharge may be present in postmenopausal women. Abdominal and pelvic examination are unremarkable, except in late cases.

There is no certain method for screening the population at risk. Outpatient endometrial sampling is useful but not foolproof.

Careful fractional diagnostic curettage and, if possible, hysteroscopy, should be carried out if this condition is suspected clinically.

Management

1. *Pre-operative evaluation* is as for carcinoma of the cervix (p. 265). Among other suggested investigations are transvaginal ultrasound, MRI or CT scan.
2. *Clinical staging* is carried out at EUA and fractional curettage.

   Stage 0: Atypical hyperplasia suspicious of malignancy
   Stage I: Carcinoma confined to the body of the uterus
   Stage Ia: Uterine cavity ⩽ 8 cm in length or only superficial myometrial invasion on histology
   Stage Ib: Uterine cavity > 8 cm in length or tumour extends through more than half of myometrial wall

   Stage I is further subdivided according to the histology:

   Grade 1: Well differentiated tumour
   Grade 2: Differentiated tumour but with partly solid areas
   Grade 3: Undifferentiated tumour or predominantly solid

   Stage II: Carcinoma involving the body and cervix
   Stage III: Carcinoma outside the uterus but not outside the true pelvis
   Stage IV: Carcinoma outside the true pelvis or involvement of the bladder or rectal mucosa
3. *Treatment*

   Stage I, Grade I: Total abdominal hysterectomy, bilateral salpingo-oophorectomy (BSO) and removal of a cuff of vagina

   Stage I, Grades 2 and 3
   Stage II } Radical hysterectomy with BSO

   Post-operative radiotherapy can be given if:

   (i) The tumour extends through more than half of the myometrial wall
   (ii) The ovaries are involved
   (iii) Growth extends to the cervix
   (iv) Pelvic lymph nodes are positive

   Stage III: Radiotherapy
   Stage IV: Radiotherapy and progestogens

Results from cytotoxic therapy are disappointing.
Pre-operative radiotherapy does not improve the prognosis and makes histological grading of the tumour more difficult.

Recurrent disease can be treated with progestogen and/or radiotherapy. Pelvic exenteration is occasionally possible and a solitary vaginal vault lesion may be excisable.

Prognosis

The 5-year survival rate is:

Stage I:	80–85%	
Grade 1:	90%	
Grade 3:	65%	
Stage II:	55–60%	(80% in best centres)
Stage III:	35–40%	(60% in best centres)
Stage IV:	< 10%	(15% in best centres)

SARCOMA OF THE UTERUS

These are rare tumours. Malignant degeneration in a leiomyoma accounts for half of them but they may arise from normal myometrium or endometrial stroma.

Leiomyosarcoma. Most patients are between 40 and 60 years of age. The commonest symptoms are abnormal vaginal bleeding and abdominal pain. A uterine mass is frequently palpable. Lymphatic spread is not common. Treatment is by total hysterectomy and bilateral salpingo-oophorectomy. Radiotherapy is relatively ineffective.

Endometrial sarcoma. Most patients are between 50 and 70 years of age. Signs, symptoms and treatment are the same as for leiomyosarcoma.

Sarcoma botryoides — a rare tumour probably of mixed mesodermal origin usually occurring in children. It is polypoidal, either single or multiple. Treatment combines chemotherapy with radiotherapy and then radical surgery (extended hysterectomy and vaginectomy).

Prognosis

The 5-year survival rate is about 45% for stage I disease and 30% in stage II.

CARCINOMA OF THE FALLOPIAN TUBE

Primary tumours of the Fallopian tube are exceedingly rare (0.3% of genital tract cancers). They tend to occur in women aged 40–60 years. The histology is papillary adenocarcinoma. The majority of patients will have had a watery vaginal discharge, and some will complain of abdominal pain. An abdominal mass may be palpable, but very few patients have all of these clinical features.

Treatment is by total hysterectomy and bilateral salpingo-oophorectomy. External radiotherapy is applied afterwards, and chemotherapy can be used in some late cases.

Five-year survival rates are between 5 and 25% reflecting the lateness of diagnosis in most case.

SUGGESTED FURTHER READING

Fox H, Buckley C H 1982 Pathology for gynaecologists. Edward Arnold, London

Malkin J C, Tindall V R 1988 Current approaches: endometrial carcinoma. Duphar Medical Relations

Tindall V R 1990 Jeffcoate's principles of gynaecology. 5th edn. Butterworth, London

Conditions of the ovary

NON-NEOPLASTIC DISTENSION CYSTS

Follicular cyst(s) ('cystic ovary')

Due to enlargement of one or more follicles which fail to rupture.

They are seldom more than 5 cm in diameter except when due to overdosage with clomiphene or HMG (see p. 194).

Often associated with:

(i) Anovulatory cycles
(ii) Fertility drugs as above
(iii) Polycystic ovary syndrome (p. 175)

The majority are symptomless

Pain (usually mild but sometimes severe) is due to rupture of or haemorrhage into the cyst. (If unilateral pain is accompanied by slight menstrual disturbance an ectopic pregnancy must be excluded.)

Management

(i) If ovarian enlargement estimated at 4 to 6 cm is found at pelvic examination carry out pelvic ultrasound. If the presumed diagnosis is a 'cystic ovary' rather than a neoplasm no immediate action is necessary. Re-examine in two weeks; a follicular cyst will usually have disappeared. If the cyst is unchanged or larger, further investigation (e.g. laparoscopy) is warranted
(ii) If discovered or confirmed by laparoscopy, the cysts can be aspirated. Laparotomy is not necessary
 Send the fluid for cytology to definitely exclude neoplasia
(iii) Treat any underlying condition

Theca–lutein cysts

A corpus luteum becomes cystic and persists in a functional state for longer than normal *or* the granulosa and theca cells of a follicular cyst become luteinised.

Characteristically, short periods of amenorrhoea are followed by heavier than usual uterine bleeding.

The endometrium is secretory.

(Haemorrhage from even a normal corpus luteum can mimic ectopic pregnancy closely.)

Multiple and sometimes moderately large theca–lutein cysts are associated with trophoblast tumours. This is due to hCG stimulation

Management

(i) Spontaneous resolution is usual
(ii) If a laparotomy is performed because of a mistaken diagnosis of ectopic pregnancy interfere with the ovary as little as possible

Endometriomatous (chocolate) cysts

Due to ovarian endometriosis (see p. 183).

OVARIAN NEOPLASMS

The incidence tends to rise with age but there is an increase in benign tumours in the fifth decade (40 to 49 years) and in malignant tumours from 50 years of age onwards.

There is an association between ovarian cancer and:

1. Nulliparity
2. Social class (mortality in class I twice that in class V).
3. Breast cancer — 50% excess of ovarian cancer has been suggested if breast cancer is (or has been) present.
4. Endometrial cancer — this relates mainly to endometrioid ovarian tumour and thecal cysts (see later)

Oral contraceptives have the same protective effect as pregnancy. There may also be a protective effect associated with mumps virus.

A carcinogenic role for particles such as asbestos or talc is unproven.

Ovarian tumours comprise 35% of all gynaecological malignancies. Although it is the sixth commonest in incidence, the ovary is the fourth commonest site for fatal malignant disease in the female, after breast, colon and lung.

Histological types and derivation

Three types of cells give rise to the vast majority of primary ovarian tumours:

1. Surface epithelium (mesothelium)
2. Germ cells
3. Gonadal stroma (sex cord mesenchyme)

They may sometimes be mixed.

Surface epithelial tumours

These tumours mimic tissues derived from the Müllerian or paramesonephric duct. They comprise:

1. Serous papillary tumours
   Benign: serous cystadenoma
   Malignant: serous cystadenocarcinoma
   They account for about 10% of ovarian neoplasms, and are bilateral in about 50% of cases. Usually unilocular with a smooth outer surface. The internal papillae may sprout through the capsule giving an impression of malignancy. The lining cells are cuboidal or columnar, resembling the epithelium of the endosalpinx
2. Mucinous tumours
   Benign: mucinous cystadenoma
   Malignant: mucinous cystadenocarcinoma
   They form 30 to 40% of ovarian neoplasms, and are often large, unilateral multilocular cysts. Loculi are lined by tall mucus-secreting columnar cells. They may be found along with a Brenner tumour (see below). Between 5 and 10% show areas of malignancy on removal.
   If the cyst ruptures the mucus-secreting cells may implant on the peritoneum and produce the rare but chronic pseudomyxomaperitonei
3. Endometrioid tumours
   These solid tumours frequently contain elements of both serous and mucinous tumours. An allegedly good prognosis when the tumour is malignant may be due to the difficulty of recognising it when it is undifferentiated. There is a definite association with endometrial carcinoma, perhaps as a result of simultaneous neoplasia in tissue of common embryonic origin
4. Clear cell ('mesonephroid') tumours
   This may be a variant for the endometrial tumour because they often co-exist
5. Brenner tumour
   It is unilateral and usually benign. It shows cords of squamous or transitional cells round a central core lined by columnar epithelium. The fibrous tissue element closely resembles that found in a fibroma (see below)
6. Fibroma
   The classification of this tumour is not easy. The tumour is often moderately large, hard and lobulated with a glistening surface. It is bilateral in about 10% of cases. The main interest of this rare tumour is its association with ascites and pleural effusion (usually right-sided) known as Meigs' syndrome. Such findings cannot therefore be presumed to be pathognomonic of advanced malignancy

Germ cell tumours
The first group arises from totipotential differentiated germ cells either from embryonic or extra-embryonic structures.

1. Teratomas — from embryonic structures
   Benign (mature tissues): dermoid cyst
   Malignant (immature tissues): teratocarcinoma
   Dermoid cysts are the commonest ovarian tumours in young women. They are usually symptomless, but torsion or rupture may produce signs and symptoms of an acute abdomen. They are bilateral in about 10% of case and seldom grow larger than 12 cm in diameter. They are lined by stratified squamous epithelium with its usual cutaneous elements — hair, sebaceous and sweat glands. Teeth, neural tissue, cartilage, alimentary and respiratory epithelium and even active thyroid tissue (struma ovarii) may be present.
   Solid teratomas may be benign but are usually malignant
2. Extra-embryonic germ cell tumours
   Choriocarcinoma
   Endodermal sinus tumour — differentiation towards yolk sac tissue. These tumours produce pregnancy-associated plasma proteins, e.g.
   choriocarcinoma — hCG (and hPL to a lesser extent)
   yolk sac — AFP
   These can be used as tumour markers in diagnosis and follow-up after treatment.
   Malignant tumours from (1) and (2) have in the past had a bad prognosis. Intensive chemotherapy is now producing better results.
3. Disgerminoma
   From undifferentiated germ cells. It is the counterpart of the seminoma in males. It is a very rare tumour arising mostly between 20 and 30 years of age. It can usually be dealt with by conservative surgery and is very radiosensitive.

Gonadal stromal tumours
The stromal cells retain a potential for differentiation into any of the cells or tissues arising from the mesenchyme of the gonad namely granulosa, theca, Leydig and Sertoli cells.
These rare tumours may therefore secrete any or all of the ovarian steroids. They tend to be classified according to morphology:
1. Granulosa — theca cell group which may produce oestrogen
   Granulosa-cell tumour — not infrequently malignant but usually of low grade
   Thecoma — fibroma
2. Sertoli–Leydig cell group (which may secrete androgens)
   Sertoli–Leydig cell tumour (androblastoma, arrhenoblastoma)
   Sertoli-cell tumour
   Leydig-cell tumour (hilus or lipoid cell tumour)
3. Mixed — elements of granulosa cell tumour and arrhenoblastoma present (gynandroblastoma)

Feminising (oestrogen-producing) tumours cause:
Precocious puberty before the menarche
Cystic glandular hyperplasia in menstruating women
Postmenopausal bleeding in older women
There is an association with endometrial carcinoma.

Masculinising (androgen-producing) tumours will initially result in defeminisation, including secondary amenorrhoea then hirsutes, enlargement of the clitoris and deepening of the voice.

Secondary ovarian tumours

Signs or symptoms referrable to the breast, stomach, large bowel and uterus must be sought.

The rare Krukenberg tumour usually results from simultaneous primary tumours in the gastrointestinal tract (particularly stomach) or breast and both ovaries.

The histology is characterised by clumps of mucus-secreting epithelial cells in stroma. The mucin compresses the nuclei of each cell to one pole producing 'signet-ring cells.'

Clinical features of ovarian tumours

The peak age incidence is between 40 and 60 years with the exception of teratomas and gonadal stromal tumour which occur at any age.

They rarely give rise to symptoms early in their course. This means that:

1. They are often found accidentally
2. If they are malignant the disease has commonly spread outside the ovary before the diagnosis is made

Abdominal swelling may be present but ignored by the patient.

Menstrual function is not usually affected (except by the rare gonadal stromal tumours).

A cyst lying in the pouch of Douglas is likely to be a dermoid.

Ovarian tumours are dull to percussion anteriorly with resonance in the flanks (cf. ascites).

Differential diagnosis

Ovarian tumour must be distinguished from a whole variety of pelvic and abdominal swellings. Among the causes which must be excluded are:

Physiological	Full bladder
	Flatus
	Faeces
	Pregnancy
	Obesity
Congenital	Uterine anomaly
	Pelvic or polycystic kidney
Traumatic	Rectus abdominis haematoma

Infective	Pyosalpinx or hydrosalpinx
	Pelvic abscess
	Appendix abscess
	Diverticulitis
	TB peritonitis
Neoplastic	Fibroids
	Tumours of colon and rectum
	Ascites
	Retroperitoneal tumour
	Mesenteric cyst
Hormonal	Non-neoplastic cysts
Mechanical	Hydronephrosis
Pregnancy-associated	Pregnancy in a uterine horn
	Ectopic pregnancy
	Corpus luteum of pregnancy

Aids to diagnosis

1. Ultrasound
2. Laparoscopy
3. Tumour markers — the results are, so far, disappointing except for the rare germ cell tumours

Clinical features in malignant versus benign tumours

1. *Age* — tumours in childhood are frequently malignant. In older women the risk of malignancy is proportional to age; 45% of tumours removed from women aged 45 years or over are malignant
2. *Pain and tenderness* — benign tumours are never painful unless complicated (see below). A sudden severe pain suggests torsion or rupture. Dull aching pain may suggest malignancy. Sacral nerve root pain is strongly suggestive of malignancy
3. *Rapidity of growth* — suggests malignancy
4. *Number of tumours*; 75% of malignant tumours are bilateral, and 15% of benign tumours are bilateral
5. *Consistency of tumours* — solid, nodular and irregular growths are more likely to be malignant
6. *Fixation* is suggestive of malignancy, but not necessarily so
7. *Ascites* is usually a sign of peritoneal metastasis (especially if the fluid is bloodstained). Remember the possibility of Meigs' syndrome
8. *Oedema* of the legs and vulva or evidence of venous obstruction are suggestive of malignancy
9. *Metastatic deposits.* Remote metastases are not common, but in advanced disease supraclavicular nodes may become enlarged. The pouch of Douglas may contain irregular deposits which can be felt on bi-manual examination. The

majority of patients with ovarian cancer present with advanced disease

Complications of ovarian cysts

1. *Torsion.* Acute or subacute pain may be accompanied by mild shock. The lower abdomen is tender with guarding and rigidity. Pelvic examination reveals a tender adnexal mass. Laparotomy is indicated and removal of the ovary usually necessary
2. *Rupture.* The signs and symptoms will vary. The contents of chocolate and dermoid cysts are extremely irritant and therefore may cause severe symptoms
3. *Haemorrhage* into or from cyst. The signs and symptoms will vary according to the degree of haemorrhage
4. *Infection.* This is not a common complication of ovarian tumours
5. *Malignant change.* This occurs mostly in serous and mucinous cystadenoma. New symptoms are not produced

Ovarian cancer screening

Several tests, singly or in combination, have been suggested for screening, e.g.:

Bimanual pelvic examination
Abdominal or vaginal ultrasound
Serum CA125 levels

No single test or combination is sufficiently specific or sensitive. On current evidence the benefit of screening is unproved.

Management of 'benign' ovarian tumours

Laparotomy must be undertaken in the presence of any ovarian swelling >5 cm diameter, particularly if it is continuing to enlarge. However, the status of the tumour will often not be certain at that crucial time.

A combination of the following features found at laparotomy may indicate (a higher risk of) malignancy:

1. The tumour is totally or partly solid
2. Bilateral tumours
3. There is fungation through the capsule (not merely papillary growths)
4. Large vessels on the tumour surface
5. Blood-stained ascites
6. Invasion of or adhesion to surrounding structures
7. Metastatic deposits

If there is real doubt, a frozen section should be asked for. In tumours known or thought to be benign the treatment depends on the age and parity of the patient.

In young women who wish to conserve reproductive capacity enucleation of the cyst (cystectomy) is carried out. Larger cysts may demand removal of the ovary. It is often prudent to bisect and biopsy the other ovary to exclude an occult tumour.

In older women past child-bearing it is customary to remove both ovaries and the uterus.

Management of early carcinoma of the ovary

All the commoner malignant tumours are considered together because the stage and histological grading of the malignancy are more important prognostic indicators than the type of tumour.

A midline or paramedian incision is required for full examination of the abdomen, particularly the diaphragm.

Accurate staging is vital.

Technique of staging

The following should be inspected and biopsied if involvement is likely or suspected:

1. Peritoneal washings for cytology
2. Parietal peritoneum
3. Omentum
4. Uterus and other ovary
5. Bladder
6. Pelvic peritoneum — biopsy if ovary is adherent
7. Bowel and its mesentery
8. Lymph nodes — para-aortic and pelvic; biopsy if possible
9. Liver — surface and substance
10. Diaphragm — both leaves

The clinical stages are as follows:

Stage I	Growth limited to the ovaries
Stage Ia:	Only one ovary involved; no ascites (sub-groups: capsule not ruptured; capsule ruptured)
Stage Ib:	Both ovaries involved; no ascites (sub-groups as above)
Stage Ic	One or both ovaries involved plus ascites or with malignant cells in peritoneal washing (sub-groups as above)
Stage IIb:	Extension to other pelvic tissues
Stage IIc:	As above with ascites or positive peritoneal washing
Stage III:	Growth involving one or both ovaries with intraperitoneal metastasis
Stage IV:	Growth involving one or both ovaries with distant metastasis

Surgery in early disease

The treatment of choice for stage I carcinoma of the ovary is bilateral salpingo-oophorectomy, hysterectomy and omentectomy.

Simple oophorectomy may be indicated for younger women

appendicectomy

with stage Ia disease (and favourable histology) who wish to preserve their reproductive capacity and who fully understand the risks.

Adjuvant therapy is not indicated for stage I disease unless:

1. The tumour is poorly differentiated
2. Ascites was present
3. The cyst was ruptured

Single-agent chemotherapy is the preferred treatment but external beam radiotherapy may be used.

Management of advanced ovarian carcinoma

Every attempt should be made to remove all macroscopic tumour.

Single-agent chemotherapy is, in general, as effective as multiple-agent treatment.

An alkylating agent (such chlorambucil, melphelan or cyclophosphamide) or cis-platinum/carboplatin can be used.

Complete remissions are possible.

Survival rates for primary ovarian carcinoma

Stage Ia:	85%
Stage Ib–IIa:	40%
Stage IIb:	25%
Stage IIc–III:	15%
Stage IV:	<5%

Second-look operations

A second-look operation, usually by laparotomy, sometimes by laparoscopy, can be carried out about 12 months after the initial operation. The examination is as described above. According to the result the clinician can:

1. Discontinue therapy
2. Resect residual disease *or*
3. Identify residual disease requiring a change in therapy

SUGGESTED FURTHER READING

Tindall V R 1990 Jeffcoate's principles of gynaecology. 5th edn. Butterworths, London

U K Co-ordinating Committee on Cancer Research 1989 Ovarian Cancer Screening

The climacteric

The *menopause* is the time at which menstruation ceases.
The *climacteric* is the transitional period during which woman's reproductive capacity ceases.
The average age at which the menopause occurs is 51 years.

PHYSICAL CHANGES OCCURRING FROM THE MENOPAUSE

Ovaries
Cortical thinning occurs and the ovaries shrink in size (some hormone synthesis persists).

Genital tract
Myometrial cells are partly replaced by fibrous tissue; endometrium is thin and atrophic. The uterus is reduced in size. Changes in the vulva and vagina are gradual over many years. The vagina becomes more smooth, narrower and less well lubricated. The pH rises and the skin of the vulva and vagina become atrophic. The labia shrink. The pelvic floor muscle becomes more lax with an increased risk of utero-vaginal prolapse.

Bladder and urethra
The epithelium thins and is more liable to infection.

Skin and breasts
The epidermis and dermis become thinner and less elastic; sebaceous and sweat gland secretion decreases. The glandular tissue of the breast atrophies, being replaced by fat.

Cardio-vascular systems
The levels of cholesterol, phospholipids and triglycerides rise and the risk of coronary artery disease gradually increases.

Skeleton
Calcium is lost from the bone at about 1% per year; gradual osteoporosis results.

SYMPTOMS ASSOCIATED WITH THE CLIMACTERIC

About half of all women have slight climacteric symptoms which last for up to a year. Another 25% seek help because of the severity of the symptoms. The remainder seem to be unaffected.

Symptoms frequently begin before the menopause. There are five groups of interlinked symptoms.

1. *Vasomotor*, e.g. hot flushes and night sweats; the aetiology is not understood; it is not merely lack of oestrogen
2. *Emotional* — e.g. lethargy, lack of concentration, irritability, aggressiveness, depression, lability of mood, anxiety
3. *Sexual* — decreased libido; dyspareunia — often due to atrophic vaginitis
4. *Urinary*, e.g. urgency and frequency of micturition — usually due to atrophic trigonitis and urethritis
5. *Musculo-skeletal* — laxity of ligaments and decreasing muscular strength may give rise to a variety of joint-related aches and pains

Management

General medical disorders (e.g. hyperthyroidism) need to be excluded.

Therapy is of three main types:

1. Hormones and other drugs
2. Treatment of related disorders e.g. obesity, hypertension
3. Psychological support

HORMONE REPLACEMENT THERAPY (HRT)

1. Cyclical oestrogen–progestogen therapy for women in whom the uterus is still present, *or*
2. Unopposed continuous oestrogen orally or by implant, in women who have had hysterectomy

Contra-indications to HRT

High risk factors include thrombo-embolism, oestrogen-dependent tumours (e.g. breast or endometrium), liver disease, and pre-existing coronary artery disease.

The presence of fibroids or a history of endometriosis are relative contra-indications.

Close observation is necessary for women taking HRT who are obese, hypertensive, diabetic, heavy smokers or have varicose veins.

Other drugs for vasomotor symptoms

Clonidine improves vasomotor symptoms for some patients.

Propranolol does not reduce hot flushes but may help tachycardia or palpitations.

Psychotropic drugs are not appropriate for purely menopausal symptoms.

Duration of treatment
Some women wish to discontinue treatment after 1 or 2 years. Other need to continue HRT for many years.

POST-MENOPAUSAL BLEEDING (PMB)

All cases must be thoroughly investigated (except perhaps for the withdrawal bleeding which occurs at the expected time in menopausal women taking HRT).
Investigations must include:

1. Complete pelvic examination
2. Cervical smear
3. Endometrial biopsy — this can often be achieved as an outpatient. If not, proceed to formal DIC.

SUGGESTED FURTHER READING

Whitehead M I 1985 The climacteric. In: Studd J (ed) Progress in obstetrics and gynaecology. Churchill Livingstone, Edinburgh, Vol 5, p 332

Preoperative assessment and management of postoperative complications in gynaecological surgery

PREOPERATIVE ASSESSMENT BEFORE MAJOR SURGERY

The correct operation must be carried out for the correct reasons. If the management suggested in outpatients is found not to be appropriate at the time of admission it must be altered accordingly or deferred for further investigation as appropriate.

Women who smoke and are scheduled to have a general anaesthetic should be advised to stop smoking several weeks before the proposed operation.

Those on the combined pill should be advised to stop several weeks before admission because of the increased risk of thrombo-embolism.

Advice about alternative contraception must be given.

Outpatient assessment must include:

1. General physical examination, including breasts, cardiac and respiratory status and BP
2. Haemoglobin and blood group estimation
3. ECG and chest X-ray, urea and electrolyte estimation in hypertensive women

Anaemia should be corrected before admission.

Obese women should be encouraged to lose weight.

Elective surgery is best avoided in the winter months for those with chronic bronchitis.

The length of time the woman should spend in hospital preoperatively must be determined by her age, fitness, general medical complications, condition for which admitted and proposed procedure.

Among the patients who require particularly careful assessment are:

1. Those with medical disorders such as cardiac disease, hypertension, diabetes mellitus or other endocrine disorders

2. Those on treatment which may affect their response to anaesthesia or surgery e.g. antihypertensives (particularly beta-blocking agents); psycho-active drugs (particularly mono- amine oxidase inhibitors); anticoagulants; systemic corticosteroids
3. The morbidly obese — this is a significant risk factor in postoperative morbidity and mortality.

Blood should be sent in good time to allow grouping and saving of serum or cross-matching depending on the extent of the surgery involved.

POSTOPERATIVE COMPLICATIONS

Any surgeon or anaesthetist must be competent to deal with the immediate hazards which may occur during an operation such as haemorrhage or cardiac failure.

Thrombo-embolism

Pelvic surgery is particularly liable to produce this complication. It is best dealt with by prophylaxis.

1. *Predisposing factors* should be eliminated as far as possible, e.g. oral contraceptive usage, obesity, varicose veins. A previous history of thrombo-embolism must be noted carefully
2. *Reduction of venous stasis.* Graded elastic stockings can be worn pre- and postoperatively by women at risk. Other methods include raising the heels from the operating table, and postoperative exercise of the calf muscles

Reduction of coagulability of blood

(i) Prophylactic subcutaneous calcium heparin 5000 units twice daily can be given either to all women over the age of 40 or to those at particular risk (e.g. past history of thrombo-embolism, troublesome varicose veins, marked obesity)

(ii) Low-molecular-weight dextran 1 litre can be infused preoperatively (this may affect cross-matching if the blood is taken after administration)

The above measures have probably reduced the overall incidence of deep-vein thrombosis but they may not have affected the incidence of fatal pulmonary embolism significantly.

Management of suspected or established thrombo-embolism

The symptoms and signs of pulmonary embolism (PE) can be missed. Typically there is pleuritic pain, haemoptysis, dyspnoea and various degrees of hypotension. It may however, present with dry cough, pyrexia, tachycardia or bronchospasm. There may be evidence of a preceding DVT.

Investigation
Chest X-ray; ECG; lung scan using ^{99}technetium^{m} (if PE is suspected); venography if DVT is suspected.

Acute therapy
Calcium heparin 15 000 units i.v. as bolus then 10 000 units 6-hourly by continuous i.v. infusion for at least 48 hours.

Longer-term therapy
Warfarin sodium 30 mg as loading dose. No more until the evening of day 2 when the correct dose is determined by the one-stage prothrombin time taken that morning. Maintain for at least 3 months.

Vault-haematoma and pelvic infection
To prevent this the following is recommended:
1. Preoperative vaginal preparation with povidone–iodine
2. Complete haemostasis during surgery
3. Adequate drainage of the pelvis
4. Prophylactic antibiotics: ampicillin and/or metronidazole for abdominal and vaginal hysterectomy

Wound haematoma and dehiscence
A transverse suprapubic incision should be used when possible but is not appropriate for management of ovarian cancer. Aseptic technique is vital. Haemostasis and closure techniques are important.

A non-absorbable or polyglycolic acid suture is preferred for closure of the rectus sheath. Drainage must be adequate.

Urinary tract complications
The incidence of *urinary infection* can be reduced by eliminating catheterisation as much as possible. The patient is asked to void urine before the pre-medication is given. A distended bladder can be emptied during the operation by syringe and needle if needs be. If continuous bladder drainage is necessary postoperatively a suprapubic catheter should be used.

Injuries to the urinary tract are preventable, but if they occur prompt recognition at the time and appropriate remedial action are appropriate. If an injury is not detected for some time after surgery it should await tissue healing and elimination of infection before repair is attempted.

Respiratory complications
A cuffed endotracheal tube must be used for all major surgery to prevent inhalation of gastric contents.

Physiotherapy should be begun preoperatively and continued postoperatively in smokers and those with respiratory complaints. Regional anaethesia may be more appropriate for some women with respiratory problems. Purulent sputum should be sent for culture, physiotherapy interrupted, and an appropriate antibiotic commenced to prevent pneumonia developing.

Index